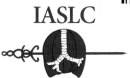

IASLC

Conquering Thoracic Cancers Worldwide

SECOND EDITION

Staging Manual in Thoracic Oncology

SECOND EDITION

Staging Manual in Thoracic Oncology

Ramón Rami-Porta, MD, Executive Editor

An International Association for the Study of Lung Cancer Publication

Editorial Rx Press

North Fort Myers, FL

International Association for the Study of Lung Cancer
Aurora, CO, USA

Executive Editor: Ramón Rami-Porta, MD
Chair, IASLC Staging and Prognostic Factors Committee
Hospital Universitari Mútua Terrassa, University of Barcelona, Terrassa, Spain

An IASLC publication published by Editorial Rx Press

Editorial Rx Press, Registered Office: North Fort Myers, FL 33917
www.editorialrxpress.com

First Editorial Rx Press Printing 2016

10 9 8 7 6 5 4 3 2

ISBN: 978-0-9832958-4-6

Chapter 1–Used with permission of the American Joint Committee on Cancer (AJCC), Chicago, Illinois. The original and primary source for this information is the AJCC Cancer Staging Manual, Seventh Edition (2010) published by Springer Science+Business Media.

Chapters 2, 4, 11, 16, 20–Used with the permission of the Union for International Cancer Control (UICC), Geneva, Switzerland. The original source for this material is the UICC TNM Classification of Malignant Tumours, 8th edition (2017), published by John Wiley & Sons, Ltd, www.wiley.com.

Chapter 5, 6, 7, 12, 13, 21– Used with the permission of the Union for International Cancer Control (UICC), Geneva, Switzerland. The original source for this material is the TNM Supplement: A Commentary on Uniform Use, 4th Edition (2012) published by John Wiley & Sons Ltd, www.wiley.com.

Chapter 23–Used with permission of the Union for International Cancer Control (UICC), Geneva, Switzerland. The original source of this material is the UICC Prognostic Factors in Cancer, 3rd Edition (2006) published by John Wiley & Sons Ltd., www.wiley.com.

Cover and interior design by Amy Boches, Biographics.

Use of the AJCC and UICC logos provided.

Dedication

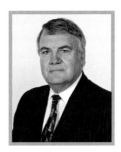

To Prof. Peter Goldstraw, MBChB, FRCS

Emeritus Professor of Thoracic Surgery,
National Heart and Lung Institute, Imperial College,
Honorary Consultant in Thoracic Surgery, Royal Brompton Hospital, London,
President (2011-2013), International Association for the Study of Lung Cancer (IASLC),
Chair (1998-2009) and Past Chair (2009-2016), IASLC Staging and Prognostic
Factors Committee

With gratitude, esteem, and respect

Acknowledgments

The International Association for the Study of Lung Cancer (IASLC) expresses its most sincere gratitude to all the investigators and their institutions around the world for their voluntary contribution to the IASLC, the International Mesothelioma Interest Group (IMIG), the International Thymic Malignancies Interest Group (ITMIG) and the Worldwide Esophageal Cancer Collaboration (WECC) staging projects. Without their collaboration and submission of their cases, the data-based revisions leading to the 8th edition of the TNM classifications of thoracic malignancies would have not been possible.

Participating Investigators and Institutions in the IASLC Lung Cancer Staging Project Database

F. Abad Cavaco and E. Ansótegui Barrera, Hospital La Fe, Valencia, Spain; J. Abal Arca and I. Parente Lamelas, Complejo Hospitalario de Ourense, Ourense, Spain; A. Arnau Obrer and R. Guijarro Jorge, Hospital General Universitario de Valencia, Valencia, Spain; D. Ball, Peter MacCallum Cancer Centre, Melbourne, Australia; G. K. Bascom, Good Samaritan Hospital, Kearney, NE, USA; A. I. Blanco Orozco and M. A. González Castro, Hospital Virgen del Rocío, Sevilla, Spain; M. G. Blum, Penrose Cancer Center, Colorado Springs, USA; D. Chimondeguy, Hospital Universitario Austral, Argentina; V. Cvijanovic, Military Medical Academy, Belgrade, Serbia; S. Defranchi, Hospital Universitario-Fundacion Favaloro, Buenos Aires, Argentina; B. de Olaiz Navarro, Hospital de Getafe, Getafe, Spain; I. Escobar Campuzano and I. Macía Vidueira, Hospital de Bellvitge, L'Hospitalet de Llobregat, Spain; E. Fernández Araujo and F. Andreo García, Hospital Universitari Germans Trias i Pujol, Badalona, Spain; K. M. Fong, Prince Charles Hospital, Brisbane, Australia; G. Francisco Corral and S. Cerezo González, Hospital La Mancha Centro, Ciudad Real, Spain; J. Freixinet Gilart, Hospital Universitario 'Dr. Negrín', Las Palmas de Gran Canaria, Spain; L. García Arangüena, Hospital Sierrallana, Torrelavega, Spain; S. García Barajas, Hospital Infanta Cristina, Badajoz, Spain; P. Girard, L'Institut Mutualiste Montsouris, Paris, France; T. Goksel, Turkish Thoracic Society, Turkey; M. T. González Budiño, Hospital General Universitario de Oviedo, Oviedo, Spain; G. González Casaurrán, Hospital Gregorio Marañón, Madrid, Spain; J. A. Gullón Blanco, Hospital San Agustín, Avilés, Spain; J. Hernández Hernández, Hospital de Ávila, Avila, Spain; H. Hernández Rodríguez, Hospital Universitario de Tenerife, Santa Cruz de Tenerife, Spain; J. Herrero Collantes, Hospital Universitario Nuestra Señora de la Candelaria, Santa Cruz de Tenerife, Spain; M. Iglesias Heras, Hospital de Ávila, Ávila, Spain; J. M. Izquierdo Elena, Hospital Nuestra Señora de Aránzazu, Donostia, Spain; E. Jakobsen, Danish Lung Cancer Registry, Denmark; S. Kostas, Athens School of Medicine, Athens, Greece; P. León Atance and A. Núñez Ares, Complejo Hospitalario de Albacete, Albacete, Spain; M. Liao, Shanghai Lung Tumor Clinical Medical Center, Shanghai, China; M. Losanovscky, Clinica y Maternidad Suizo Argentina, Buenos Aires, Argentina; G. Lyons, Hospital Britanico de Buenos Aires, Buenos Aires, Argentina; R. Magaroles and L. De Esteban Júlvez, Hospital Joan XXIII, Tarragona. Spain; M. Mariñán Gorospe, Hospital de San Pedro de Logroño, Logroño, Spain; B. McCaughan and C. Kennedy, University of Sydney, Sydney, Australia; R. Melchor Íñiguez, Fundación Jiménez Díaz, Madrid, Spain; L. Miravet Sorribes, Hospital La Plana, Castellón, Spain; S. Naranjo Gozalo and C. Álvarez de Arriba, Hospital Universitario Marqués de Valdecilla, Santander, Spain; M. Núñez Delgado, Hospital de Meixoeiro, Vigo, Spain; J. Padilla Alarcón and J. C. Peñalver Cuesta, Instituto Valenciano de Oncología, Valencia, Spain; J. S. Park, Samsung Medical Center, Seoul, South Korea; H. Pass, New York University Langone Medical Center and Cancer Center, New York, USA; M. J. Pavón Fernández, Hospital 'Severo Ochoa', Leganés, Spain; M. Rosenberg, Alexander Fleming Institute and Hospital de Rehabilitación Respiratoria, Buenos Aires, Argentina; E. Ruffini, University of Torino, Torino , Italy; V. Rusch, Memorial Sloan-Kettering Cancer Center, New York, USA; J. Sánchez de Cos Escuín, Hospital de Cáceres, Cáceres, Spain; A. Saura Vinuesa, Hospital de Sagunto, Sagunto, Spain; M. Serra Mitjans, Hospital Universitari Mútua Terrassa, Terrassa, Spain; T.E. Strand, Cancer Registry of Norway, Norway; D. Subotic, Clinical Centre of Serbia, Belgrade, Serbia; S. Swisher, M.D. Anderson Cancer Center (MDACC), Houston, USA; R. Terra, University of Sao Paulo Medical Center, Sao Paulo, Brazil; C. Thomas, Mayo Clinic Rochester, Rochester, MN, USA; K. Tournoy, University Hospital Ghent, Belgium; P. Van Schil, Antwerp University Hospital, Edegem (Antwerp), Belgium; M. Velasquez, Fundacion Clinica Valle del Lili, Cali, Colombia; Y. L. Wu, Guangdong General Hospital, Guangzhou, China; K. Yokoi, Japanese Joint Committee for Lung Cancer Registry, Osaka, Japan.

Participating Investigators and Institutions in the IASLC Mesothelioma Staging Project Database

H. Asamura, Keio University, Japan; H. Batirel, Marmara University, Turkey; A. Bille and U. Pastorino, Istituto Nazionale dei Tumori, Italy; S. Call Caja, Mutua Terrassa University Hospital, Spain; A. Cangir, Ankara University School of Medicine, Turkey; S. Cedres, Vall d'Hebron University Hospital, Spain; J. Friedberg, University of Pennsylvania - Penn-Presbyterian Medical Center, USA; F. Galateau-Sallé, University

Hospital Center (CHU) of Caen (MesoNAT Registry), France; S. Hasagawa, Hyogo College of Medicine, Japan; K. Kernstine, University of Texas Southwestern Medical Center, USA; H. Kindler, University of Chicago, USA; B. McCaughan, Univeristy of Sydney, Australia; T. Nakano, Hyogo College of Medicine, Japan; A. Nowak, Sir Charles Gairdner Hospital, Australia; C. Atinkaya Ozturk, Sureyyapasa Training and Research Hospital, Turkey; H. Pass, NYU Langone Medical Center, USA; M. de Perrot, Toronto General Hospital and Princess Margaret Hospital, University of Toronto, Canada; F. Rea, University of Padova, Italy; D. Rice, The University of Texas MD Anderson Cancer Center, USA; R. Rintoul, Papworth Hospital NHS Foundation Trust, UK; E. Ruffini, University of Torino, Italy; V. Rusch, Memorial Sloan-Kettering Cancer Center, USA; L. Spaggiari and D. Galetta, European Institute of Oncology, Italy; K. Syrigos, University of Athens Oncology Unit, Greece; C. Thomas, Mayo Clinic Rochester, USA; J. van Meerbeeck, Univeristy Hospital Antwerp and University Hospital Ghent, Belgium; J. Vansteenkiste, University Hospital Leuven, Belgium; W. Weder and I. Opitz, UniversitätsSpital Zürich, Switzerland; M. Yoshimura, Hyogo Cancer Center, Japan.

Participating Investigators and Institutions in the IASLC/ITMIG Thymic Malignancies Staging Project Database

S. Call Caja, Hospital Universitari Mútua Terrassa, Terrassa, Spain; U. Ahmad and F. Detterbeck, Yale Cancer Center, New Haven, CT, USA; N. Girard, Louis Pradel Hospital, Lyon, France; S. J. Haam, Gangnam Severance Hospital, Seoul, Korea; M. K. Bae, Severance Hospital, Seoul, Korea; D.R. Gomez and E. M. Marom, MD Anderson Cancer Center, Houston, TX, USA; P. Van Schil, Antwerp University Hospital, Antwerp, Belgium; P. Ströbel, University Medical Center Göttingen, Göttingen, Germany; A. Marx, University Medical Center Mannheim, Mannheim, Germany; S. Saita, Azienda Ospedaliero-Universitaria Policlinico V. Emanuele, Catania, Italy; H. Wakelee, Stanford University, Stanford, CA, USA; L. Bertolaccini, Thoracic Surgery, Azienda Ospedaliera S.Croce e Carle, Cuneo, Italy; E. Vallières, Swedish Cancer Institute, Seattle, WA, USA; W. Scott and S. Su, Fox Chase Cancer Center, Philadelphia, PA, USA; B. Park and J. Marks, Hackensack University Medical Center, Hackensack, NJ, USA; S. Khella, Penn Presbyterian Medical Center, Philadelphia, PA, USA; R. Shen, Mayo Clinic Rochester, Rochester, MN, USA; M. Rosenberg, Alexander Fleming Institute, Buenos Aires, Argentina; M. Rosenberg, Maria Ferrer Institute, Buenos Aires, Argentina; V. Tomulescu, Fundeni Clinical Institute, Bucharest, Romania; J. Huang, Memorial Sloan Kettering Cancer Center, New York, NY, USA; C. Foroulis, AHEPA University Hospital, Aristotle University Medical School, Thessaloniki, Greece; L. Lang-Lazdunski and A. Billè, Guy's & St Thomas Hospital, London, UK; J.G. Maessen and M. Keijzers, Maastricht University Medical Centre, Maastricht, Netherlands; H. van Veer, University Hospitals Leuven, Belgium; C. Wright, Massachusetts General

Hospital, Boston, MA, USA; M. Marino and F. Facciolo, Regina Elena National Cancer Institute, Rome, Italy; G. Palmieri and C. Buonerba, Università Degli Studi di Napoli Federico II, Napoli, Italy; M. Ferguson, University of Chicago, Chicago, IL, USA; G. Marulli, University of Padua, Padua, Italy; M. Lucchi, University of Pisa, Pisa, Italy; P. Loehrer, Indiana University Simon Cancer Center, IN, USA; M. Kalkat, Birmingham Heartlands Hospital, Birmingham, UK; K. Rohrberg and G Daugaard, Rigshospitalet, University Hospital of Copenhagen, Copenhagen, Denmark; A. Toker and S. Erus, Istanbul Medical University, Istanbul, Turkey; M. Kimmich, Klinik Schillerhoehe, Gerlingen, Germany; A. Brunelli and M. Refai, Ospedali Riuniti, Ancona, Italy; A. Nicholson and E. Lim, Royal Brompton Hospital / Harefield NHS Foundation Trust, London, UK; I. K. Park, Seoul National Hospital, Seoul, Korea; J. Wagner and B. Tieu, Oregon Health and Science University, Portland, Oregon, USA; W. Fang and J. Zhang, Shanghai Chest Hospital, Jiaotong University Medical School, Shanghai, China; Z. Yu, Tianjin Medical University Cancer Hospital, Tianjin, China; Y. Han, Sichuan Cancer Hospital, Chengdu, China; Y. Li, Henan Cancer Hospital, Zhengzhou, China; K. Chen, Beijing University Cancer Hospital, Beijing, China; G. Chen, Shanghai Pulmonary Hospital, Tongji University, Shanghai, China; M. Okumura, Osaka University, Osaka, Japan; Y. Fujii, Nagoya City University, Aichi, Japan; H. Asamura, National Cancer Center Hospital, Tokyo, Japan; K. Nagai, National Cancer Center Hospital East, Chiba, Japan; J. Nakajima, University of Tokyo, Tokyo, Japan; N. Ikeda, Tokyo Medical University, Tokyo, Japan; S. Haraguchi, Nippon Medical School, Tokyo, Japan; T. Onuki, Tokyo Women's Medical University, Tokyo, Japan; K. Suzuki, Juntendo University, Tokyo, Japan; I. Yoshino, Chiba University, Chiba, Japan; M. Tsuchida, Niigata University, Niigata, Japan; S. Takahashi, Shizuoka Cancer Center, Shizuoka, Japan; K. Yokoi, Nagoya University, Aichi, Japan; M. Hanyuda, Aichi Medical University, Aichi, Japan; H. Niwa, Seirei Mikatahara General Hospital, Shizuoka, Japan: H. Date, Kyoto University, Kyoto, Japan; Y. Maniwa, Kobe University, Hyogo, Japan; S. Miyoshi, Okayama University, Okayama, Japan; K. Kondo, Tokushima University, Tokushima, Japan; A. Iwasaki, Fukuoka University, Fukuoka, Japan; T. Okamoto, Kyusyu University, Fukuoka, Japan; T. Nagayasu, Nagasaki University, Nagasaki, Japan; F. Tanaka, University of Occupational and Environmental Health, Fukuoka, Japan; M. Suzuki, Kumamoto University, Kumamoto, Japan; K. Yoshida, Shinsyu University, Nagano, Japan; Y. Okuma and H. Horio, Tokyo Metropolitan Cancer and Infectious Diseases Center Komagome Hospital, Tokyo, Japan; A. Matsumura, Kinki Chuo Chest Medical Center, Osaka, Japan; M. Higashiyama, Osaka Medical Center for Cancer and Cardiovascular Diseases, Osaka, Japan; H. Suehisa, Shikoku Cancer Center, Ehime, Japan; T. Onuki, Tsuchiura Kyodo Hospital, Ibaragi, Japan; Y. Sano, Ehime University, Ehime, Japan; K. Kondo, Hokkaido Cancer Center, Hokkaido, Japan; K. Al Kattan, King Khaled Unversity Hospital, Riyadh, Saudi Arabia; R. Cerfolio, University of Alabama, Birmingham, AL, USA;

C. Gebitekin, Uludag University School of Medicine, Bursa, Turkey; D. Gómez de Antonio, Hospital Universitario Puerta de Hierro Majadahonda, Madrid, Spain; K. H. Kernstine, University of Texas, Southwestern Medical Center and School of Medicine (SW), Dallas, USA; N. Altorki, The New York Hospital, Cornell Medical Centre, New York, USA; N. Novoa, Salamanca University Hospital, Salamanca, Spain; E. Ruffini and P. L. Filosso, University of Torino, Torino, Italy; S. Saita, University of Catania, Catania, Italy; M. Scarci, Papworth Hospital NHS Foundation Trust, Papworth Everard, Cambridge, UK; L. Voltolini, Università di Siena, Siena, Italy; W. Weder, University Hospital, Zurich, Switzerland; W. Zurek, Medical University of Gdansk, Gdansk, Poland; A. Arame, Hopital Europeen Georges-Pompidou and Hopital Laennec, Paris, France; C. Casadio, Chirurgia Toracica, Novara, Italy; P. Carbognani, Università di Parma, Parma, Italy; G. Donati, Ospedale di Aosta, Aosta, Italy; S. Keshavjee, University of Toronto, Toronto, Canada; W. Klepetko and B. Moser, Medical University of Vienna, Vienna, Austria; C. Lequaglie, Thoracic Surgery, Rionero in Vulture, Italy; M. Liberman, Centre Hospitalier de l'Université de Montréal, Montréal, Canada; M. Mancuso, Ospedale Alessandria, Alessandria, Italy; M. Nosotti, Policlinico, Milan, Italy; L. Spaggiari, Istituto Europeo di Oncologia (IEO), Milan, Italy; P. A. Thomas, Hôpital Nord - Université de la Méditerranée, Marseille, France; E. Rendina, University La Sapienza, Ospedale Sant' Andrea, Rome, Italy; F. Venuta and M. Anile, Policlinico Umberto I, Rome, Italy; J. Schützner, Teaching Hospital Motol, Prague, Czech Republic; G. Rocco, Pascale Institute, Napoli, Italy.

Participating Investigators and Institutions in the Worldwide Esophageal Cancer Collaboration Staging Project Database

K. N. Chen, Beijing Cancer Hospital, Peking University, Beijing, China; T. W. Rice and E. H. Blackstone, Cleveland Clinic, Cleveland, OH, USA; C. Apperson-Hansen, Case Western Reserve University, Cleveland, OH, USA; B. P.L. Wijnhoven , J. van Lanschot and S. Lagarde, Erasmus Medical Center, Rotterdam, The Netherlands; J-F. Liu, Fourth Hospital of Hebei Medical University, Shijiazhuang, Hebei, China; W. J. Scott and D. Edmondson, Fox Chase Cancer Center, Philadelphia, PA, USA; R. Burger, Groote Schuur Hospital, University of Cape Town, Cape Town, South Africa; A. R. Davies and J. Zylstra, Guy's & St. Thomas' Hospitals, London, UK; J. V. Räsänen, J. A. Salo and Y. Sundstrom, Helsinki University Hospital, Helsinki, Finland; M. Pera, Hospital Universitario del Mar, Barcelona, Spain; X. B. D'Journo, Hôpital Nord, Marseille; France; K. A. Kesler, Indiana University Medical Center, Indianapolis, IN, USA; W. L. Hofstetter, A. Correa and S. G. Swisher, University of Texas MD Anderson Hospital, Houston, TX, USA; M. S. Allen, Mayo Clinic, Rochester, MN, USA; C. E. Denlinger, Medical University of South Carolina, Charleston, SC, USA; V. W. Rusch, Memorial Sloan-Kettering Cancer Center, New York, NY, USA; B. M. Smithers, D. Gotley, A. Barbour and I. Thomson, University of Queensland, Princess

Alexandra Hospital, Brisbane, Australia; S. M. Griffin and J. Shenfine, University of Newcastle upon Tyne, Newcastle upon Tyne, UK; P. H. Schipper and J. G. Hunter, Oregon Health & Science University, Portland, OR, USA; W. H. Allum, Royal Marsden Hospital, London, UK; W. (Vincent) Fang, Shanghai Chest Hospital, Shanghai, China; G. E. Darling, Toronto General Hospital, Toronto, ON, Canada; T. E.M.R. Lerut and P. R. Nafteux, University Zeikenhuizen Leuven, Leuven, Belgium; R. van Hillegersberg, University Medical Center Utrecht, Utrech, The Netherlands; R. J. Cerfolio, University of Alabama at Birmingham, Birmingham, AL, USA; L. Durand and R. De Antón, Hospital de Clinicas, University of Buenos Aires, Buenos Aires, Argentina; M. K. Ferguson, The University of Chicago, Department of Surgery, Chicago, IL, USA; S. Law, University of Hong Kong Medical Center, Queen Mary Hospital, Hong Kong, China; M. B. Orringer and B. L. Marshall, University of Michigan, Ann Arbor, MI, USA; A. Duranceau and S. Howson, University of Montreal, Montreal, Quebec, Canada; J. D. Luketich, A. Pennathur and K. Lovas, University of Pittsburgh Medical Center, Pittsburgh, PA, USA; T. J. Watson, University of Rochester, Rochester, NY, USA; I. Cecconello, University of São Paulo, São Paulo, Brazil; L-Q. Chen, West China Hospital of Sichuan University, Chengdu, Sichuan, China.

"Nought may endure but mutability!"

—Percy B. Shelley

Contents

Contents

Contributors

Editorial Committee
Executive Editor
Ramón Rami-Porta

Associate Editors
Hisao Asamura
Frank C. Detterbeck
Peter Goldstraw
Thomas W. Rice
Valerie W. Rusch

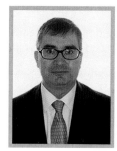
Ramón Rami-Porta

Members

Alex A. Adjei (Editor-in -Chief, Journal of Thoracic Oncology), Mayo Clinic, Rochester, MN, USA.

Hisao Asamura (Chair-Elect and Chair, N-Descriptors Subcommittee of the IASLC Staging and Prognostic Factors Committee, Japan Lung Cancer Society Liaison), Keio University, Tokyo, Japan.

Eugene H. Blackstone (Member of the Advisory Board of the IASLC Oesophageal Cancer Domain of the IASLC Staging and Prognostic Factors Committee, and the Worldwide Esophageal Cancer Collaboration), Cleveland Clinic, Cleveland, OH, USA.

James Brierley (Co-Chair, Union for International Cancer Control TNM Committee and UICC Liaison), Princess Margaret Cancer Centre/University Health Network, University of Toronto, Toronto, ON, Canada.

David Carbone (IASLC President), Ohio State's Comprehensive Cancer Center-James Cancer Hospital and Research Institute, Columbus, OH, USA.

John Crowley (Chief of Strategic Alliances), Cancer Research And Biostatistics, Seattle, WA, USA.

Frank C. Detterbeck (Chair, Thymic Malignancies Domain and Chair, Methodology and Validation Subcommittee of the IASLC Stating and Prognostic Factors Committee, and International Thymic Malignancies Interest Group Liaison), Yale University, New Haven, CT, USA.

Wilfried E. E. Eberhardt (Chair, M-Descriptors Subcommittee of the IASLC Staging and Prognostic Factors Committee), West German Cancer Centre, University Hospital, Ruhrlandklinik, Univesity Duisburg-Essen, Essen, Germany.

Pier Luigi Filosso (Member of the Advisory Board of the Thymic Malignancies Domain of the IASLC Staging and Prognostic Factors Committee), University of Torino, Torino, Italy.

Dorothy Giroux (Biostatistician), Cancer Research And Biostatistics, Seattle, WA, USA.

Peter Goldstraw (Past-President IASLC, Past-Chair IASLC Staging and Prognostic Factors Committee), Royal Brompton Hospital, Imperial College, London, UK.

Mary K. Gospodarowicz (Immediate Past President of the UICC, Co-Chair of the UICC TNM Core Group), Princess Margaret Hospital/University Health Network, University of Toronto, Toronto, Canada.

Fred R. Hirsch (CEO, IASLC and Board of Directors Liaison), University of Colorado Health Sciences, Denver, Colorado, USA.

Eng-Siew Koh, Princess Margaret Hospital/University Health Network, University of Toronto, Toronto, Canada.

Andrew G. Nicholson (Chair, Small Cell Lung Cancer Subcommittee of the IASLC Staging and Prognostic Factors Committee), Royal Brompton Hospital and Harefield NHS Foundation Trust and Imperial College, London, UK.

Brian O'Sullivan (Chair, UICC Prognostic Factors Committee, Member of the UICC TNM Core Group), Princess Margaret Hospital/University Health Network, University of Toronto, Toronto, Canada.

Harvey I. Pass (Member of the Advisory Board of the IASLC Mesothelioma Domain of the IASLC Staging and Prognostic Factors Committee), New York University, New York, NY, USA.

Ramón Rami-Porta (Chair, IASLC Staging and Prognostic Factors Committee and Chair, Lung Cancer Domain and T-Descriptors Subcommittee), Hospital Universitari Mútua Terrassa, University of Barcelona, and Centros de Investigación Biomédica en Red de Enfermedades Respiratorias (CIBERES) Lung Cancer Group, Terrassa, Barcelona, Spain.

Thomas W. Rice (Chair, Carcinoma of the Oesophagus Domain of the IASLC Staging and Prognostic Factors Committee, and World Wide Esophageal Collaboration Liaison), Cleveland Clinic, Cleveland, OH, USA.

Valerie W. Rusch (Chair, Mesothelioma Domain of the IASLC Staging and Prognostic Factors Committee, and American Joint Committee on Cancer Liaison), Memorial Sloan-Kettering Cancer Center, New York, NY, USA.

Nagahiro Saijo (IASLC President 2007-2009), Former Deputy Director National Cancer Center East, Chiba, Executive Officer of the Japanese Society of Medical Oncology, Japan.

Jean-Paul Sculier (Chair, Prognostic Factors Subcommittee of the IASLC Staging and Prognostic Factors Committee), Institut Jules Bordet, Brussels, Belgium.

Lynn Shemanski (Senior Biostatistician), Cancer Research And Biostatistics, Seattle, WA, USA.

William D. Travis (Chair, Neuroendocrine Tumours Subcommittee of the IASLC Staging and Prognostic Factors Committee), Memorial Sloan-Kettering Cancer Center, New York, NY, USA.

Ming S. Tsao (Chair, Biologic Factors Subcommittee of the IASLC Staging and Prognostic Factors Committee), The Princess Margaret Cancer Centre, Toronto, Ontario, Canada.

IASLC Staging and Prognostic Factors Committee

Peter Goldstraw, Past-Chair, Royal Brompton Hospital and Imperial College, London, United Kingdom; Ramón Rami-Porta, Chair, Hospital Universitari Mútua Terrassa, Terrassa, Spain; Hisao Asamura, Chair-Elect, Keio University, Tokyo, Japan; David Ball, Peter MacCallum Cancer Centre, Melbourne, Australia; David Beer, University of Michigan, Ann Arbor, MI, United States of America (USA); Ricardo Beyruti, University of Sao Paulo, Brazil; Vanessa Bolejack, Cancer Research And Biostatistics, Seattle, WA, USA; Kari Chansky, Cancer Research And Biostatistics, Seattle, WA, USA; John Crowley, Cancer Research And Biostatistics, Seattle, WA, USA; Frank C. Detterbeck, Yale University, New Haven, CT, USA; Wilfried Ernst Erich Eberhardt, West German Cancer Centre, University Hospital, Ruhrlandklinik, University Duisburg-Essen, Essen, Germany; John Edwards, Northern General Hospital, Sheffield, United Kingdom; Françoise Galateau-Sallé, Centre Hospitalier Universitaire, Caen, France; Dorothy Giroux, Cancer Research And Biostatistics, Seattle, WA, USA; Fergus Gleeson, Churchill Hospital, Oxford, United Kingdom; Patti Groome, Queen's Cancer Research Institute, Kingston, Ontario, Canada; James Huang, Memorial Sloan-Kettering Cancer Center, New York, NY, USA; Catherine Kennedy, University of Sydney, Sydney, Australia; Jhingook Kim, Samsung Medical Center, Seoul, Korea; Young Tae Kim, Seoul National University, Seoul, South Korea; Laura Kingsbury, Cancer Research And Biostatistics, Seattle, WA, USA; Haruhiko Kondo, Kyorin University Hospital, Tokyo, Japan; Mark Krasnik, Gentofte Hospital, Copenhagen, Denmark; Kaoru Kubota, Nippon Medical School Hospital, Tokyo, Japan; Toni Lerut, University Hospitals, Leuven, Belgium; Gustavo Lyons, British Hospital, Buenos Aires, Argentina; Mirella Marino, Regina Elena National Cancer Institute, Rome, Italy; Edith M. Marom, MD Anderson Cancer Center, Houston, TX,

USA; Jan van Meerbeeck, Antwerp University Hospital, Edegem (Antwerp), Belgium; Alan Mitchell, Cancer Research And Biostatistics, Seattle, WA, USA; Takashi Nakano, Hyogo College of Medicine, Hyogo, Japan; Andrew G. Nicholson, Royal Brompton and Harefield NHS Foundation Trust and Imperial College, London, United Kingdom; Anna Nowak, University of Western Australia, Perth, Australia; Michael Peake, Glenfield Hospital, Leicester, United Kingdom; Thomas W. Rice, Cleveland Clinic, Cleveland, OH, USA; Kenneth Rosenzweig, Mount Sinai Hospital, New York, NY, USA; Enrico Ruffini, University of Torino, Torino, Italy; Valerie W. Rusch, Memorial Sloan-Kettering Cancer Center, New York, NY, USA; Nagahiro Saijo, National Cancer Center Hospital East, Chiba, Japan; Paul Van Schil, Antwerp University Hospital, Edegem (Antwerp), Belgium; Jean-Paul Sculier, Institut Jules Bordet, Brussels, Belgium; Lynn Shemanski, Cancer Research And Biostatistics, Seattle, WA, USA; Kelly Stratton, Cancer Research And Biostatistics, Seattle, WA, USA; Kenji Suzuki, Juntendo University, Tokyo, Japan; Yuji Tachimori, National Cancer Center, Tokyo, Japan; Charles F. Thomas Jr, Mayo Clinic, Rochester, MN, USA; William D. Travis, Memorial Sloan-Kettering Cancer Center, New York, NY, USA; Ming S. Tsao, The Princess Margaret Cancer Centre, Toronto, Ontario, Canada; Andrew Turrisi, Sinai Grace Hospital, Detroit, MI, USA; Johan Vansteenkiste, University Hospitals, Leuven, Belgium; Hirokazu Watanabe, National Cancer Center Hospital, Tokyo, Japan; Yi-Long Wu, Guangdong General Hospital, Guangzhou, People's Republic of China.

T Coding and Size Measurement in Preinvasive and Lepidic Adenocarcinoma *ad hoc* Workgroup

William D. Travis (chair), Hisao Asamura, Alex Bankier, Mary Beth Beasley, Frank Detterbeck, Douglas B. Flieder, Jin Mo Goo, Heber MacMahon, David Naidich, Andrew Nicholson, Charles A. Powell, Mathias Prokop, Ramón Rami-Porta, Valerie Rusch, Paul Van Schil, Yasushi Yatabe.

Multiple Pulmonary Sites of Involvement *ad hoc* Workgroup

Frank Detterbeck (chair), Douglas A. Arenberg, Hisao Asamura, Vanessa Bolejack, John Crowley, Jessica S. Donington, Wilbur A. Franklin, Nicolas Girard, Edith M. Marom, Peter J. Mazzone, Andrew G. Nicholson, Valerie W. Rusch, Lynn T. Tanoue, William D. Travis.

Advisory Board of the IASLC Mesothelioma Domain

Paul Baas, The Netherlands Cancer Institute, Amsterdam, The Netherlands; Jeremy Erasmus, MD Anderson Cancer Center, Houston, TX, USA; Seiki Hasegawa, Hyogo College of Medicine, Hyogo, Japan; Kouki Inai, Hiroshima University Postgraduate School, Hiroshima, Japan; Kemp Kernstine, City of Hope, Duarte, CA, USA; Hedy Kindler, The University of Chicago Medical Center, Chicago, IL, USA; Lee Krug,

Memorial Sloan-Kettering Cancer Center, New York, NY, USA; Kristiaan Nackaerts, University Hospitals, Leuven, Belgium; Harvey Pass, New York University, NY, USA; David Rice, MD Anderson Cancer Center, Houston, TX, USA.

Advisory Board of the IASLC Thymic Malignancies Domain

Conrad Falkson, Queen's University, Ontario, Canada; Pier Luigi Filosso, University of Torino, Italy; Giuseppe Giaccone, Georgetown University, Washington, DC, USA; Kazuya Kondo, University of Tokushima, Tokushima, Japan; Marco Lucchi, University of Pisa, Pisa, Italy; Meinoshin Okumura, Osaka University, Osaka, Japan.

Advisory Board of the IASLC Oesophageal Cancer Domain

Eugene Blackstone, Cleveland Clinic, OH, USA.

Preface to the Second Edition

By David P. Carbone, MD, PhD, IASLC President, 2015-2017, and
Fred R. Hirsch, MD, PhD, Chief Executive Officer

The staging of lung cancer and other thoracic malignancies is important for the treatment decisions. The Union for International Cancer Control/American Joint Committee on Cancer/International Association for the Study of Lung Cancer (UICC/AJCC/IASLC) Staging Classification is used all over the world and the IASLC is proud of launching the 8th Edition of the International Staging of Thoracic Malignancies. While the previous 7th Edition of the staging system was focusing on lung cancer, the new 8th Edition also includes staging of thymus cancers, malignant pleural mesothelioma, and carcinoma of the oesophagus. The new staging system is based on about 100.000 cases collected by international multidisciplinary investigators from all geographical regions of the world.

For the second consecutive time, the IASLC has been in charge to provide the UICC and the AJCC with data-based recommendations to revise the TNM classification of thoracic malignancies. Both institutions have accepted the IASLC recommendations and incorporated them in their respective 8th Edition staging manuals published in 2016.

The IASLC staging project has been performed by the IASLC Staging and Prognostic Factors Committee under the leadership of Dr. Ramón Rami-Porta, MD, Spain. This project could not be performed without the generous unrestricted support from Lilly Oncology, USA.

The IASLC is proud to serve the international oncological community and thanks the UICC and the AJCC for entrusting it with such challenging and intellectually rewarding responsibility. It is our hope that the 8th Edition of the Staging Classification will be a useful tool for further research and will serve in the daily lung cancer clinic to the benefit for the many patients with lung cancer around the world.

Preface to the First Edition

By Nagahiro Saijo, MD, IASLC President, 2007-2009

The International Association for the Study of Lung Cancer (IASLC) is proud to present the details of the IASLC/International Union Against Cancer (UICC)/American Joint Committee on Cancer (AJCC) Revised Staging Classification for Lung Cancer in this Manual. The IASLC is the largest world-wide professional organization solely dedicated to reducing the worldwide burden of lung cancer. The International Staging Classification for Lung Cancer provides the basis for assigning prognosis and treatment selection for patients with lung cancer. Thus, its importance cannot be overemphasized, especially as we develop new methods of staging. These new methods include clinical procedures such as computed tomographic (CT) scans and CT/positron emission tomographic (PET) scans and new pathologic procedures such as endobronchial ultrasound (EBUS)-guided biopsies and video-assisted thoracic surgery (VATS) biopsies. The IASLC recognizes that the staging classification will be most valuable and accurate if it is based on large numbers of cases carefully collected and analyzed. We are indebted to the diligent efforts of the IASLC Staging Committee chaired by Dr. Peter Goldstraw and whose members are listed in the Manual; the diligent efforts of the Cancer Research And Biostatistics (CRAB) office headed by Dr. John Crowley; the support of the IASLC Board of Directors whose members are also listed in the Manual; the financial support of Eli Lilly and Company and the support of the UICC and the AJCC to create a staging classification supported worldwide. We thank these individuals and organizations for their support and trust the revised staging classification will improve the outcome for lung cancer patients and their families.

Introduction

By Ramón Rami-Porta, MD, PhD, FETCS, Executive Editor
Chair, IASLC Staging and Prognostic Factors Committee

The second phase of the International Association for the Study of Lung Cancer (IASLC) Staging Projects culminates with the publication of the second edition of the IASLC *Staging Manual in Thoracic Oncology* and the IASLC *Staging Handbook in Thoracic Oncology*. During these eight years since 2009, new datasets have been designed to register data on patients with lung cancer, malignant pleural mesothelioma and thymic tumours, and a memorandum of understanding was agreed with Dr. Thomas W. Rice, from the Cleveland Clinic, Cleveland, OH, USA, for an educational association to promote and disseminate the tumour, node and metastasis (TNM) classification of oesophageal cancer based on a new database of cases registered by the Worldwide Esophageal Cancer Collaboration (WECC). The IASLC also has worked in collaboration with the International Thymic Malignancies Interest Group (ITMIG) regarding the staging data of these tumours and with the International Mesothelioma Interest Group (IMIG), as well as with other organizations interested in the staging of malignant tumours, such as the European Society of Thoracic Surgeons, the Japanese Association for Research on the Thymus, and the Japanese Joint Committee for Lung Cancer Registry, among others. These entities and many institutions around the world sent data from their databases to Cancer Research And Biostatistics (CRAB) whose statisticians analysed and interpreted in close association with the members of the IASLC Staging and Prognostic Factors Committee and with the members of the newly created Advisory Boards. The Advisory Boards consist of additional specialists who contribute their work and expertise to the IASLC Staging Projects. From the functional point of view, the members of the IASLC Staging and Prognostic Factors Committee were distributed in four different domains according to their areas of interest: Lung Cancer Domain, Malignant Pleural Mesothelioma Domain, Thymic Tumours Domain and Oesophageal Cancer Domain. (Appendix) Each domain has a chair, who is the link with the members of the Advisory Boards, and may have several subcommittees for specific tasks. (Figures 1 and 2)

The amount of collected data is huge. Table 1 shows the number of evaluable patients used for the revision of the TNM classifications of lung cancer, malignant pleural mesothelioma and oesophageal carcinoma, and for the development of an

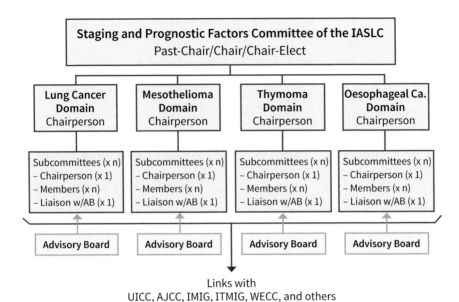

Figure 1. Structure of the International Association for the Study of Lung Cancer Staging and Prognostic Factors Committee. Notes: n: number; w: with; AB: Advisory Board; UICC: Union for International Cancer Control; AJCC: American Joint Committee on Cancer; IMIG: International Mesothelioma Interest Group; ITMIG: International Thymic Malignancies Interest Group; WECC: Worldwide Esophageal Cancer Collaboration.

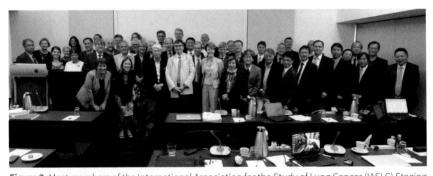

Figure 2. Most members of the International Association for the Study of Lung Cancer (IASLC) Staging and Prognostic Factors Committee met in Sydney, Australia, on October 25 and 26, 2013, prior to the 15th World Conference on Lung Cancer, to discuss the latest analyses of the IASLC database and decide on the recommendations for changes. This picture was taken at the end of the sessions on October 25, 2013.

internationally agreed TNM classification for thymic malignancies. The analyses of the lung cancer database produced a series of original articles describing the characteristics of the database[1], the analyses, findings and recommendations for changes on the T[2], the N[3], and the M[4] components of the classification, as well as those for the revision of the stages.[5] In addition, the recommended changes, based on the analyses of non-small cell lung cancer, were tested in the population of patients with small cell lung cancer. They were found to be useful in this cancer although the survival curves reflect the different natural history of small cell lung cancer and its worse prognosis.[6] The issue of how to classify lung cancers with multiple lesions was thoroughly discussed in four original papers on different patterns of disease: simultaneous second primaries,[7] separate tumour nodules,[8] multiple adenocarcinomas presenting as ground glass opacities on computed tomography and

Table 1. Number of Evaluable Patients Used for Revision of the TNM Classifications of Thoracic Malignancies.

Tumour	Number of Evaluable Patients
Lung cancer*	77,156
Malignant pleural mesothelioma*	2,460
Thymic malignancies**	8,145
Oesophageal cancer***	22,654

* Registered by the International Association for the Study of Lung Cancer (IASLC) and analysed by Cancer Research And Biostatistics (CRAB).
** Registered by the International Thymic Malignancies Interest Group and the IASLC, and analysed by CRAB.
*** Registered by the World Wide Esophageal Cancer Collaboration and analysed at the Cleveland Clinic, Cleveland, OH, USA.

showing lepidic features on pathologic examination,[9] and adenocarcinoma with pneumonic pattern.[9] A succinct paper summarises the rules for classification and provides concise information on the criteria to classify these lesions at clinical and pathologic staging.[10] One additional article deals with the newly incorporated tumours into the TNM classification -adenocarcinoma *in situ* and minimally invasive adenocarcinoma- and how to code them in the 8th edition of the TNM classification of lung cancer.[11] Finally, another article discusses in detail the methodological aspects of the different analyses conducted for the 8th edition.[12]

Although more than a dozen classifications of thymic malignancies had been proposed during the past few decades, none was considered official or incorporated into the staging manuals of the American Joint Committee on Cancer and the Union for International Cancer Control. For the first time in the history of anatomic staging, a data-based, internationally and multidisciplinary agreed classification will be part of the 8th edition of the TNM classification of malignant tumours. This thymic classification is, indeed, the first TNM-based internationally approved classification for this tumour site. The analyses of the IASLC/ITMIG database comprising more than 8,000 evaluable patients generated a series of original articles on the T[13] and the N and M components,[14] as well as on the stages[15] that have informed the proposed classification for the 8th edition staging manuals. A new lymph node map for exclusive use in thymic malignancies also has been proposed,[16] together with a revision of the mediastinal compartments.[17]

The analyses of the first IASLC mesothelioma database pointed out some limitations of the TNM classification.[18] Therefore, a call for the submission of more cases was launched resulting in the registration of 2,460 evaluable cases. Their analyses have generated four original articles, one on the database itself,[19] one on the T component,[20] another on the N component,[21] and another on the M component and stage grouping.[22] Not all limitations have been solved, but changes in the T and the N components, and in the stages have been suggested. In addition, an article on recommendations for uniform definitions of surgical procedures based on an IASLC/IMIG consensus was published,[23] as well as an article on prognostic factors.[24]

For the second consecutive time, the WECC database has been used to revise the TNM classification of oesophageal carcinoma. The initial one, used to inform the 7th edition of the classification, consisted of 4,627 patients who had undergone oesophageal resection with no induction therapy. Important innovations of this classification were the unification of the classification of oesophageal and oesoph-ago-gastric junction cancers, and the introduction of non-anatomical parameters, such as cell type, histopathologic grade and tumour location, to arrange stage groupings. For the 8th edition, the WECC has data on 22,654 patients and, among these, there are patients whose tumours were clinically staged, pathologically staged and pathologically staged after induction therapy. The analyses of these three populations of patients have been reported in three articles that inform the 8th edition of the TNM classification of oesophageal cancer and oesophago-gastric junction.[25, 26, 27]

I would like to thank Prof. Peter Goldstraw, Past-Chair of the IASLC Staging and Prognostic Factors Committee. Far from retiring to an easy chair, he has actively participated in the development of all activities that have led to the 8th edition of the TNM classification of thoracic malignancies, sharing his knowledge, experi-ence, common sense, diplomacy, political correctness and time, and contributing the most complex article in the series, i.e., the lung cancer stages article.[5] Ms. Deb Whippen, our publisher from Editorial Rx Press, already published the first edition of the IASLC *Staging Manual in Thoracic Oncology*[28] and the IASLC *Staging Handbook in Thoracic Oncology*,[29] has managed the production of their second edition. I thank her for her professionalism, enthusiasm, continuous availability and thoughtful suggestions. Dr. Aletta Anne Frazier, a radiologist by profession and a skillful medical illustrator, was kind enough to accept again our invitation to contribute her beauti-ful figures to the atlases of the different thoracic malignancies. I thank her for her dedication and good taste, and for devoting many hours of her time to the IASLC Staging Projects. It has been delightful to discuss with her over the phone the best options to illustrate the many categories of the four tumours included in the IASLC staging books. Nothing would have been possible without the data from our many contributors around the world. Their generosity is overwhelming. All are mentioned in the Acknowledgment section and I wholeheartedly thank them for their time, dedication and support. Ms. Dolores Martínez, Secretary to our Service of Thoracic Surgery, and Ms. Pat Vigues Frantzen, my Personal Assistant, have paid attention to every detail and have made my life much easier in so many ways that I cannot thank them enough. Finally, I would like to thank Dr. Fred Hirsch, IASLC CEO, IASLC presidents for this phase of the IASLC Staging Projects, Drs. David Gandara, Peter Goldstraw, Tony Mok and David Carbone, as well as all the IASLC Board Members, for their continuous support to the activities of the IASLC Staging and Prognostic Factors Committee.

As with the first edition, the second edition of the IASLC *Staging Manual in Thoracic Oncology* and the IASLC *Staging Handbook in Thoracic Oncology* has been produced in collaboration with the Union for International Cancer Control and the American Joint Committee on Cancer. Both institutions have granted us permission to reprint key chapters from their own books, which ensures uniformity in the three manuals. Their cooperation is much appreciated.

The IASLC Staging Projects, conceived in 1996 in London, during the International Workshop on Intrathoracic Staging, under the leadership of Prof. Peter Goldstraw and the sponsorship of the IASLC,[30] have already spanned for 20 years. After these two decades of continuous hard work, it is clear that the era of data-based revisions of the TNM classification of thoracic malignancies is consolidated. The work is not finished, though. The challenge of the combination of anatomic elements and non-anatomic elements, especially molecular markers, to construct prognostic groups and improve individualized prognosis will be the core activity of the third phase of the IASLC Staging Projects 2017-2024 that will be led by Dr. Hisao Asamura as Chair of the IASLC Staging and Prognostic Factors Committee. We count, once more, on the data sent by our colleagues around the world to make this third phase, leading to the 9th edition of the TNM classification of thoracic malignancies, a scientific success and a useful contribution to our patients.

References

1. Rami-Porta R, Bolejack V, Giroux DJ et al. The IASLC Lung Cancer Staging Project: the new database to inform the eighth edition of the TNM classification of lung cancer. *J Thorac Oncol* 2014; 9: 1618-1624.
2. Rami-Porta R, Bolejack V, Crowley J et al. The IASLC Lung Cancer Staging Project: proposals for the revisions of the T descriptors in the forthcoming 8th edition of the TNM classification for lung cancer. *J Thorac Oncol* 2015; 10: 990-1003.
3. Asamura H, Chansky K, Crowley J et al. The IASLC Lung Cancer Staging Project: proposals for the revisions of the N descriptors in the forthcoming 8th edition of the TNM classification for lung cancer. *J Thorac Oncol* 2015; 10: 1675-1684.
4. Eberhardt WEE, Mitchell A, Crowley J et al. The IASLC Lung Cancer Staging Project: proposals for the revisions of the M descriptors in the forthcoming 8th edition of the TNM classification for lung cancer. *J Thorac Oncol* 2015; 10: 1515-1522.
5. Goldstraw P, Chansky K, Crowley J et al. The IASLC Lung Cancer Staging Project: proposals for the revision of the stage grouping in the forthcoming (8th) edition of the TNM classification of lung cancer. *J Thorac Oncol* 2016; 11: 39-51.

6. Nicholson AG, Chansky K, Crowley J et al. The IASLC Lung Cancer Staging Project: proposals for the revision of the clinical and pathologic staging of small cell lung cancer in the forthcoming eighth edition of the TNM classification for lung cancer. *J Thorac Oncol* 2016; 11: 300-311.

7. Detterbeck FC, Franklin WA, Nicholson AG et al. The IASLC Lung Cancer Staging Project: proposed criteria to distinguish separate primary lung cancers from metastatic foci in patients with two lung tumors in the forthcoming eighth edition of the TNM classification·for lung cancer. *J Thorac Oncol* 2016; 11: 651-665.

8. Detterbeck FC, Bolejack V, Arenberg DA et al. The IASLC Lung Cancer Staging Project: proposals for the classification of lung cancer with separate tumor nodules in the forthcoming eighth edition of the TNM classification for lung cancer. *J Thorac Oncol* 2016; 11: 681-692.

9. Detterbeck FC, Marom EM, Arenberg DA et al. The IASLC Lung Cancer Staging Project: proposals for the application of TNM staging rules to lung cancer presenting as multiple nodules with ground glass or lepidic features or a pneumonic-type of involvement in the forthcoming eighth edition of the TNM classification. *J Thorac Oncol* 2016; 11: 666-680.

10. Detterbeck FC, Nicholson AG, Franklin WA et al. The IASLC Lung Cancer Staging Project: proposals for revisions of the classification of lung cancers with multiple pulmonary sites of involvement in the forthcoming eighth edition of the TNM classification. *J Thorac Oncol* 2016; 11: 639-650.

11. Travis WD, Asamura H, Bankier A et al. The IASLC Lung Cancer Staging Project: proposals for coding T categories for subsolid nodules and assessment of tumor size in part-solid tumors in the forthcoming eighth edition of the TNM classification of lung cancer. *J Thorac Oncol* 2016; 11: 1204-1223.

12. Detterbeck F, Groome P, Bolejack V et al. The IASLC Lung Cancer Staging Project: methodology and validation used in the development of proposals for revision of the stage classification of non-small cell lung cancer in the forthcoming (eighth) edition of the TNM classification of lung cancer. *J Thorac Oncol* 2016; 11: 1433-1446.

13. Nicholson AG, Detterbeck FC, Marino M et al. The IASLC/ITMIG Thymic Epithelial Tumors Staging Project: proposals for the T component for the forthcoming (8th) edition of the TNM classification of malignant tumors. *J Thorac Oncol* 2014; 9 (suppl 2); s73-s80.

14. Kondo K, Van Schil P, Detterbeck FC at al. The IASLC/ITMIG Thymic Epithelial Tumors Staging Project: proposals for the N and M components for the forthcoming (8th) edition of the TNM classification of malignant tumors. *J Thorac Oncol* 2014; 9 (suppl 2): s81-s87.

15. Detterbeck FC, Stratton K, Giroux D et al. The IASLC/ITMIG Thymic Epithelial Tumors Staging Project: proposals for an evidence-based stage classification system for the forthcoming (8th) edition of the TNM classification of malignant tumors. *J Thorac Oncol* 2014; 9 (suppl 2): s65-s72.

16. Bhora FY, Chen DJ, Detterbeck FC et al. The ITMIG/IASLC Thymic Epithelial Tumors Staging Project: a proposed lymph node map for thymic epithelial tumors in the forthcoming 8th edition of the TNM classification of malignant tumors. *J Thorac Oncol* 2014; 9 (suppl 2): s88-s96.

17. Carter BW, Tomiyama N, Bhora FY et al. A modern definition of mediastinal compartments. *J Thorac Oncol* 2014; 9 (suppl 2): s97-s101.

18. Rusch VW, Giroux D, Kennedy C et al. Initial analysis of the International Association for the Study of Lung Cancer Mesothelioma database. *J Thorac Oncol* 2012; 7: 1631-1639.

19. Pass H, Giroux D, Kennedy C et al. The IASLC Mesothelioma database: improving staging of a rare disease through international participation. *J Thorac Oncol* 2016; in press.

20. Nowak AK, Chansky K, Rice DC et al. The IASLC Mesothelioma Staging Project: proposals for revisions of the T descriptors in the forthcoming eighth edition of the TNM classification for mesothelioma. *J Thorac Oncol* 2016; in press.

21. Rice D, Chansky K, Nowak A et al. The IASLC Mesothelioma Staging Project: proposals for revisions of the N descriptors in the forthcoming eighth edition of the TNM classification for malignant pleural mesothelioma. *J Thorac Oncol* 2016; in press.

22. Rusch VW, Chansky K, Kindler HL et al. The IASLC Malignant Pleural Mesothelioma Staging Project: proposals for the M descriptors and for the revision of the TNM stage groupings in the forthcoming (eighth) edition of the TNM classification for mesothelioma. *J Thorac Oncol* 2016; in press.

23. Rice D, Rusch V, Pass H et al. Recommendations for uniform definitions of surgical techniques for malignant pleural mesothelioma: a consensus report of the International Association for the Study of Lung Cancer International Staging Committee and the International Mesothelioma Interest Group. *J Thorac Oncol* 2011; 6: 1304-1312.
24. Pass HI, Giroux D, Kennedy C et al. Supplementary prognostic variables for pleural mesothelioma: a report from the IASLC Staging Committee. *J Thorac Oncol* 2014; 9: 856-864.
25. Rice TW, Apperson-Hansen C, DiPaola C et al. Worldwide Esophageal Cancer Collaboration: clinical staging data. *Dis Esophagus* 2016; 7: 707-714.
26. Rice TW, Chen L-Q, Hofstetter WL et al. Worldwide Esophageal Cancer Collaboration: pathologic staging data. *Dis Esophagus* 2016; 7: 724-733.
27. Rice TW, Lerut TEMR, Orringer MB et al. Worldwide Esophageal Cancer Collaboration: neoadjuvant pathologic staging data. *Dis Esophagus* 2016; 7: 715-723.
28. Goldstraw P, ed. IASLC *Staging Manual in Thoracic Oncology*. Editorial Rx Press, Orange, FL, USA; 2009.
29. Goldstraw P, ed. IASLC *Staging Handbook in Thoracic Oncology*. Editorial Rx Press, Orange, FL, USA; 2009.
30. Goldstraw P. Report on the international workshop on intrathoracic staging. London, October 1996. *Lung Cancer* 1997; 18: 107-111.

Appendix. Members and Structure of the IASLC Staging and Prognostic Factors Committee

Past-chair: Peter Goldstraw
Chair: Ramón Rami-Porta
Chair-elect: Hisao Asamura

LUNG CANCER DOMAIN
Chair: Ramón Rami-Porta

T Descriptors Subcommittee:
Ramón Rami-Porta (chair), David Ball, Vanessa Bolejack, John Crowley, Dorothy J. Giroux, Jhingook Kim, Gustavo Lyons, Thomas Rice, Kenji Suzuki, Charles F. Thomas Jr, William D. Travis, Yi-Iong Wu

N Descriptors Subcommittee:
Hisao Asamura (chair), David Ball, Kari Chansky, John Crowley, Peter Goldstraw, Valerie Rusch, Paul Van Schil, Johan Vansteenkiste, Hirokazu Watanabe, Yi-Iong Wu, Marcin Zielinski

M Descriptors Subcommittee:
Wilfried Eberhardt (chair), Kari Chansky, John Crowley, Young Tae Kim, Haruhiko Kondo, Alan Mitchell, Andrew Turrisi

Validation and Methodology Subcommittee:
Patti Groome (chair 2010-15), Frank Detterbeck (chair 2015-7), Vanessa Bolejack, John Crowley, Catherine Kennedy, Mark Krasnik, Michael Peak

Prognostic Factors Subcommittee:
Jean-Paul Sculier (chair), Kari Chansky, John Crowley, Dorothy J. Giroux, Fergus Gleeson, Jan van Meeerbeeck

Neuroendocrine Tumours Subcommittee:
William D. Travis (chair), Hisao Asamura, Kari Chansky, John Crowley, Dorothy J. Giroux

Small Cell Lung Cancer Subcommittee:
Andrew Nicholson (chair), Ricardo Beyruti, Kari Chansky, John Crowley, Kouru Kubota, Andrew Turrisi

Biologic Factors Subcommittee:
Ming S. Tsao (chair), David G. Beer, John Crowley, Yi-Iong Wu

T Coding and Size Measurement in Preinvasive and Lepidic Adenocarcinoma **ad hoc** *Workgroup:*
William D. Travis (chair), Hisao Asamura, Alex Bankier, Mary Beth Beasley, Frank Detterbeck, Douglas B. Flieder, Jin Mo Goo, Heber MacMahon, David Naidich, Andrew Nicholson, Charles A. Powell, Mathias Prokop, Ramón Rami-Porta, Valerie Rusch, Paul Van Schil, Yasushi Yatabe

Multiple Pulmonary Sites of Involvement **ad hoc** *Workgroup:*
Frank Detterbeck (chair), Douglas A. Arenberg, Hisao Asamura, Vanessa Bolejack, John Crowley, Jessica S. Donington, Wilbur A. Franklin, Nicolas Girard, Edith M. Marom, Peter J. Mazzone, Andrew G. Nicholson, Valerie W. Rusch, Lynn T. Tanoue, William D. Travis

MALIGNANT PLEURAL MESOTHELIOMA DOMAIN
Chair: Valerie Rusch
Hisao Asamura, John Crowley, John G. Edwards, Françoise Galateau- Sallé, Dorothy J. Giroux, Catherine Kennedy, Jan van Meerbeeck, Takashi Nakano, Anna Nowack, K. E. Rosenzweig, William Travis, Johan Vansteenkiste

Mesothelioma Advisory Board:
Liaison with the Malignant Pleural Mesothelioma Domain: Valerie Rusch
Members: Paul Baas, Seiki Hasegawa, Jeremy Erasmus, Kouki Inai, Kemp Kernstein, Hedy Kindler, Lee Krug, Kristiaan Nackaerts, Harvey Pass, David Rice

THYMIC MALIGNANCIES DOMAIN
Chair: Frank Detterbeck
Hisao Asamura, John Crowley, Dorothy Giroux, James Huang, Jhingook Kim, Mirella Marino, Edith Marom, Anderew Nicholson, Enrico Ruffini, Paul Van Schil

Thymic Malignancies Advisory Board:
Liaison with the Thymic Malignancies Domain: Frank Detterbeck
Members: Conrad Falkson, Pier Luigi Filosso, Giuseppe Giaccone, Kazuya Kondo, Mario Lucchi, Meinoshin Okumura

OESOPHAGEAL CARCINOMA DOMAIN
Chair: Thomas Rice
John Crowley, Toni Lerut, Yuji Tachimori

Oesophageal Carcinoma Advisory Board:
Liaison with the Oesophageal Carcinoma Domain: Thomas Rice
Member: Eugene Blackstone

PART I

GENERAL

Executive Editor's Note: *One of the purposes of the TNM classification is "to give some indication of prognosis". This chapter, contributed by the American Joint Committee on Cancer (AJCC), provides an overview of the statistical principles and methodologies used to assess prognosis. The strengths and pitfalls inherent in each analytical method are highlighted to show the importance of choosing the correct statistical tool in each situation.*

Acknowledgment: *Used with permission of the American Joint Committee on Cancer (AJCC), Chicago, Illinois. The original and primary source for this information is in Edge SB, Byrd DR, Compton CC, Fritz AG, Greene FL, Trotti III A, eds. AJCC Cancer Staging Manual, Seventh Edition (2010) published by Springer Science+Business Media.*

1

Cancer Survival Analysis

Analysis of cancer survival data and related outcomes is necessary to assess cancer treatment programs and to monitor the progress of regional and national cancer control programs. The appropriate use of data from cancer registries for outcomes analyses requires an understanding of the correct application of appropriate quantitative tools and the limitations of the analyses imposed by the source of data, the degree to which the available data represent the population, and the quality and completeness of registry data. In this chapter the most common survival analysis methodology is illustrated, basic terminology is defined, and the essential elements of data collection and reporting are described. Although the underlying principles are applicable to both, the focus of this discussion is on the use of survival analysis to describe data typically available in cancer registries rather than to analyze research data obtained from clinical trials or laboratory experimentation. Discussion of statistical principles and methodology will be limited. Persons interested in statistical underpinnings or research applications are referred to textbooks that explore these topics at length.[1-7]

Basic Concepts

A *survival rate* is a statistical index that summarizes the probable frequency of specific outcomes for a group of patients at a particular point in time. A *survival curve* is a summary display of the pattern of survival rates over time. The basic concept is simple. For example, for a certain category of patient, one might ask what proportion is likely to be alive at the end of a specified interval, such as 5 years. The greater the proportion surviving, the lower the *risk* for this category of patients. Survival analysis, however, is somewhat more complicated than it first might appear. If one were to measure the length of time between diagnosis and death or record the vital status when last observed for every patient in a selected patient group, one might be tempted to describe the survival of the group as the proportion alive at the end of the period under investigation. This simple measure is informative only if all of the patients were observed for the same length of time.

In most real situations, not all members of the group are observed for the same amount of time. Patients diagnosed near the end of the study period are more likely to be alive at last contact and will have been followed for less time than those diagnosed earlier. Even though it was not possible to follow these persons as long as the others, their survival might eventually prove to be just as long or longer. Although we do not know the complete survival time for these individuals, we do know a minimum survival time (time from diagnosis to last known contact date), and this information is still valuable in estimating survival rates. Similarly, it is usually not possible to know the outcome status of all of the patients who were in the group at the beginning. People may be lost to follow-up for many reasons: they may move, change names, or change physicians. Some of these individuals may have died and others could be still living. Thus, if a survival rate is to describe the outcomes for an entire group accurately, there must be some means to deal with the fact that different people in the group are observed for different lengths of time and that for others, their vital status is not known at the time of analysis. In the language of survival analysis, subjects who are observed until they reach the end-point of interest (e.g., recurrence or death) are called *uncensored cases*, and those who survive beyond the end of the follow-up or who are lost to follow-up at some point are termed *censored* cases.

Two basic survival procedures that enable one to determine overall group survival, taking into account both censored and uncensored observations, are the life table method and the Kaplan–Meier method.[8,9] The life table method was the first method generally used to describe cancer survival results, and it came to be known as the actuarial method because of its similarity to the work done by actuaries in the insurance industry. It is most useful when data are only available in grouped categories as described in the next section. The Kaplan–Meier estimate utilizes individual survival times for each patient and is preferable when data are available in this form.

The specific method of computation, that is, life table or Kaplan–Meier, used for a specific study should always be clearly indicated in the report to avoid any confusion associated with the use of less precise terminology. Rates computed by different methods are not directly comparable, and when the survival experiences of different patient groups are compared, the different rates must be computed by the same method.

The concepts of survival analysis are illustrated in this chapter. These illustrations are based on data obtained from the public-use files of the National Cancer

Institute's Surveillance, Epidemiology, and End Results (SEER) Program. The cases selected are a 1% random sample of the total number for the selected sites and years of diagnosis. Follow-up of these patients continued through the end of 1999. Thus, for the earliest patients, there can be as many as 16 years of follow-up, but for those diagnosed at the end of the study period, there can be as little as 1 year of follow-up. These data are used both because they are realistic in terms of the actual survival rates they yield and because they encompass a number of cases that might be seen in a single large tumour registry over a comparable number of years. They are intended only to illustrate the methodology and concepts of survival analysis. SEER results from 1973 to 1997 are more fully described elsewhere.[10] These illustrations are not intended and should not be used or cited as an analysis of patterns of survival in breast and lung cancer in the USA.

The Life Table Method

The life table method involves dividing the total period over which a group is observed into fixed intervals, usually months or years. For each interval, the proportion surviving to the end of the interval is calculated on the basis of the number known to have experienced the endpoint event (e.g., death) during the interval and the number estimated to have been at risk at the start of the interval. For each succeeding interval, a cumulative survival rate may be calculated. The cumulative survival rate is the probability of surviving the most recent interval multiplied by the probabilities of surviving all of the prior intervals. Thus, if the percent of the patients surviving the first interval is 90% and is the same for the second and third intervals, the cumulative survival percentage is 72.9% ($0.9 \times 0.9 \times 0.9 = 0.729$).

Results from the life table method for calculating survival for the breast cancer illustration are shown in Figure 1.1. Two-thousand eight-hundred nineteen (2,819) patients diagnosed between 1983 and 1998 were followed through 1999. Following the life table calculation method for each year after diagnosis, the 1-year survival rate is 95.6%. The 5-year cumulative survival rate is 76.8%. At 10 years, the cumulative survival is 61.0 %.

The lung cancer data show a much different survival pattern (Figure 1.2). At 1 year following diagnosis, the survival rate is only 41.8%. By 5 years it has fallen to 12.0%, and only 6.8% of lung cancer patients are estimated to have survived for 10 years following diagnosis. For lung cancer patients the *median survival time* is 10.0 months. Median survival time is the point at which half of the patients have experienced the endpoint event and half of the patients remain event-free. If the cumulative survival does not fall below 50% it is not possible to estimate median survival from the data, as is the case in the breast cancer data.

In the case of breast cancer, the 10-year survival rate is important because such a large proportion of patients live more than 5 years past their diagnosis.

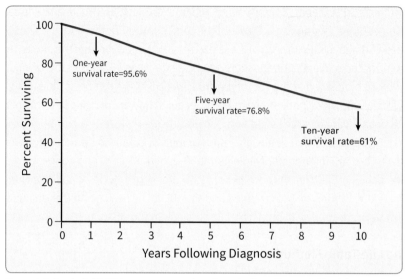

Figure 1.1. Survival of 2,819 breast cancer patients from the Surveillance, Epidemiology, and End Results Program of the National Cancer Institute, 1983-1998. Calculated by the life table method.

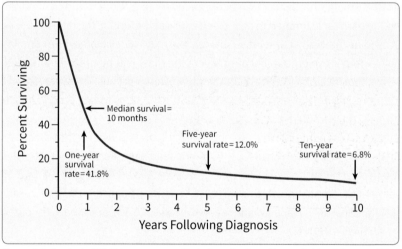

Figure 1.2. Survival of 2,347 lung cancer patients from the Surveillance, Epidemiology, and End Results Program of the National Cancer Institute, 1983-1998. Calculated by the life table method.

The 10-year time frame for lung cancer is less meaningful because such a large proportion of this patient group dies well before that much time passes.

An important assumption of all actuarial survival methods is that censored cases do not differ from the entire collection of uncensored cases in any systematic manner that would affect their survival. For example, if the more recently diagnosed cases in Figure 1.1, that is, those who were most likely not to have died yet, tended to be detected with earlier-stage disease than the uncensored cases or if they were treated differently, the assumption about comparability of censored and uncensored cases would not be met, and the result for the group as a whole would be inaccurate. Thus, it is important, when patients are included in a life table analysis, that one be reasonably confident that differences in the amount of information available about survival are not related to differences that might affect survival.

The Kaplan–Meier Method

If individual patient data are available, these same data can be analyzed using the Kaplan–Meier method.[9] It is similar to the life table method but calculates the proportion surviving to each point that a death occurs, rather than at fixed intervals. The principal difference evident in a survival curve is that the stepwise changes in the cumulative survival rate appear to occur independently of the intervals on the "Years Following Diagnosis" axis. Where available, this method provides a more accurate estimate of the survival curve.

Patient-, Disease-, and Treatment-Specific Survival

Although overall group survival is informative, comparisons of the overall survival between two groups often are confounded by differences in the patients, their tumours, or the treatments they received. For example, it would be misleading to compare the overall survival depicted in Figure 1.1 for the sample of all breast cancer cases with the overall survival for a sample of breast cancer patients who were diagnosed with more advanced disease, whose survival would be presumed to be poorer. The simplest approach to accounting for possible differences between groups is to provide survival results that are specific to the categories of patient, disease, or treatment that may affect results. In most cancer applications, the most important variable by which survival results should be subdivided is the stage of disease. Figure 1.3 shows the *stage-specific* 5-year survival curves of the same breast cancer patients described earlier. These data show that breast cancer patient survival differs markedly according to the stage of the tumour at the time of diagnosis.

Almost any variable can be used to subclassify survival rates, but some are more meaningful than others. For example, it would be possible to provide season-of-diagnosis-specific (i.e., spring, summer, winter, and fall) survival rates, but the season of diagnosis probably has no biologic association with the length of a breast cancer patient's survival. On the other hand, the race-specific and age-specific survival rates shown in Figures 1.4 and 1.5 suggest that both of these variables are related to breast cancer survival. Caucasians have the highest survival rates and African-Americans the lowest. In the case of age, these data suggest that only the oldest patients experience poor survival and that it would be helpful to consider the effects of other causes of death that affect older persons using adjustments to be described.

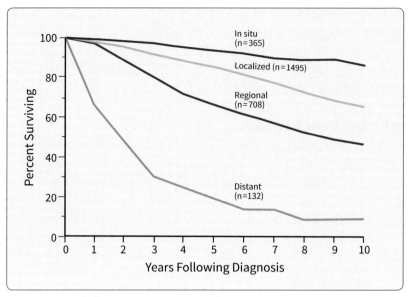

Figure 1.3. Survival of 2,819 breast cancer patients from the Surveillance, Epidemiology, and End Results Program of the National Cancer Institute, 1983-1998. Calculated by the life table method and stratified by historic stage of disease. Note: Excludes 119 patients with unknown stage of disease. SEER uses extent of disease (EOD) staging.

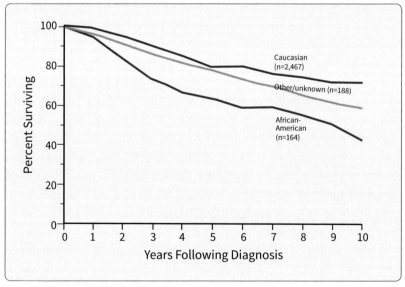

Figure 1.4. Survival of 2,819 breast cancer patients from the Surveillance, Epidemiology, and End Results Program of the National Cancer Institute, 1983-1998. Calculated by the life table method and stratified by race.

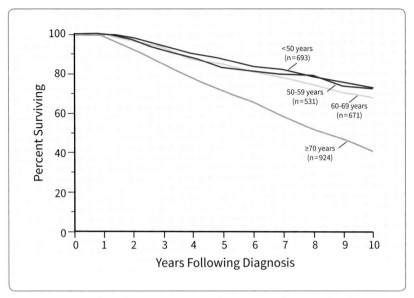

Figure 1.5. Survival of 2,819 breast cancer patients from the Surveillance, Epidemiology, and End Results Program of the National Cancer Institute, 1983-1998. Calculated by the life table method and stratified by age at diagnosis.

Although the factors that affect survival may be unique to each type of cancer, it has become conventional that a basic description of survival for a specific cancer should include stage-, age-, and race-specific survival results. Treatment is a factor by which survival is commonly subdivided, but it must be kept in mind that selection of treatment is usually related to other factors that exert influence on survival. For example, in cancer care the choice of treatment is often dependent on the stage of disease at diagnosis. Comparison of survival curves by treatment is most appropriately accomplished within the confines of randomized clinical trials.

Cause-Adjusted Survival Rate

The survival rates depicted in the illustrations account for all deaths, regardless of cause. This is known as the *observed survival rate*. Although observed survival is a true reflection of total mortality in the patient group, we frequently are interested in describing mortality attributable only to the disease under investigation. In the past, this was most often calculated using the *cause-adjusted survival rate*, defined as the proportion of the initial patient group that escaped death due to a specific cause (e.g., cancer) if no other cause of death was operating. This technique requires that reliable information on cause of death is available and makes an adjustment for deaths due to causes other than the disease under study. This was accomplished by treating patients who died without the disease of interest as censored observations.

Competing Risks/Cumulative Incidence

The treatment of deaths from other causes as censored is controversial, since statistical methods used in survival analysis settings assume that censoring is independent of outcome. This means that if the patient was followed longer, one could eventually observe the outcome of interest. This makes sense for patients lost to follow-up (if we located them, we might eventually observe their true survival time). However, if a patient dies due to another cause, we will never observe their death due to the cancer of interest. Estimation of the adjusted rate as described previously does not appropriately distinguish between patients who are still alive at last known contact date and those known to have died from another cause. These latter events are called *competing risks*.

When competing risks are present, an alternative to the Kaplan–Meier estimate is the cumulative incidence method. This technique is similar to the Kaplan–Meier estimate in its treatment of censored observations and is identical to the Kaplan–Meier estimate if there are no competing risks. However, in the presence of competing risks, the other causes of death are handled in a different manner.[11]

Relative Survival

Information on cause of death is sometimes unavailable or unreliable. Under such circumstances, it is not possible to compute a *cause*-adjusted survival rate. However, it is possible to adjust partially for differences in the risk of dying from causes other than the disease under study. This can be done by means of the *relative survival rate*, which is the ratio of the observed survival rate to the expected rate for a group of people in the general population similar to the patient group with respect to race, sex, and age. The relative survival rate is calculated using a procedure described by Ederer et al.[12]

The relative survival rate represents the likelihood that a patient will not die from causes associated specifically with the cancer at some specified time after diagnosis. It is always greater than the observed survival rate for the same group of patients. If the group is sufficiently large and the patients are roughly representative of the population of the USA (taking race, sex, and age into account), the relative survival rate provides a useful estimate of the probability of escaping death from the specific cancer under study. However, if reliable information on cause of death is available, it is preferable to use the *cause*-adjusted rate. This is particularly true when the series is small or when the patients are largely drawn from a particular socioeconomic segment of the population. Relative survival rates may be derived from life table or Kaplan–Meier results.

Regression Methods

Examining survival within specific patient, disease, or treatment categories is the simplest way of studying multiple factors possibly associated with survival. This approach, however, is limited to factors into which patients may be broadly grouped. This approach does not lend itself to studying the effects of measures that vary on an interval scale. There are many examples of interval variables in cancer, such as age, number of positive nodes, cell counts, and laboratory marker values. If the patient population were to be divided up into each interval value, too few subjects would be in each analysis to be meaningful. In addition, when more than one factor is considered, the number of curves that result provides so many comparisons that the effects of the factors defy interpretation.

Conventional multiple regression analysis investigates the joint effects of multiple variables on a single outcome, but it is incapable of dealing with censored observations. For this reason, other statistical methods are used to assess the relationship of survival time to a number of variables simultaneously. The most commonly used is the Cox proportional hazards regression model.[13] This model provides a method for estimating the influence of multiple covariates on the survival distribution from data that include censored observations. Covariates are the multiple factors to be studied in association with survival. In the Cox proportional hazards regression model, the covariates may be categorical variables such as race, interval measures such as age, or laboratory test results.

Specifics of these methods are beyond the scope of this chapter. Fortunately, many readily accessible computer packages for statistical analysis now permit the methods to be applied quite easily by the knowledgeable analyst. Although much useful information can be derived from multivariate survival models, they generally require additional assumptions about the shape of the survival curve and the nature of the effects of the covariates. One must always examine the appropriateness of the model that is used relative to the assumptions required.

Standard Error of a Survival Rate

Survival rates that describe the experience of the specific group of patients are frequently used to generalize to larger populations. The existence of true population values is postulated, and these values are estimated from the group under study, which is only a sample of the larger population. If a survival rate was calculated from a second sample taken from the same population, it is unlikely that the results would be exactly the same. The difference between the two results is called the sampling variation (chance variation or sampling error). The *standard error* is a measure of the extent to which sampling variation influences the computed survival rate. In repeated observations under the same conditions, the true or population survival rate will lie within the range of two standard errors on either side of the computed rate approximately 95 times in 100. This range is called the *95% confidence interval*.

Comparison of Survival Between Patient Groups

In comparing survival rates of two patient groups, the statistical significance of the observed difference is of interest. The essential question is, "What is the probability that the observed difference may have occurred by chance?" The standard error of the survival rate provides a simple means for answering this question. If the 95% confidence intervals of two survival rates do not overlap, the observed difference would customarily be considered statistically significant, that is, unlikely to be due to chance. This latter statement is generally true, although it is possible for a formal statistical test to yield a significant difference even with overlapping confidence intervals. Moreover, comparisons at any single time point must be made with care; if a specific time (5 years, for example) is known to be of interest when the study is planned, such a comparison may be valid; however, identification of a time based on inspection of the curves and selection of the widest difference make any formal assessment of difference invalid.

It is possible that the differences between two groups at each comparable time of follow-up do not differ significantly but that when the survival curves are considered in their entirety, the individual insignificant differences combine to yield a significantly different pattern of survival. The most common statistical test that examines the whole pattern of differences between survival curves is the *log rank test*. This test equally weights the effects of differences occurring throughout the follow-up and is the appropriate choice for most situations. Other tests weight the differences according to the numbers of persons at risk at different points and can yield different results depending on whether deaths tend more to occur early or later in the follow-up.

Care must be exercised in the interpretation of tests of statistical significance. For example, if differences exist in the patient and disease characteristics of two treatment groups, a statistically significant difference in survival results may primarily reflect differences between the two patient series, rather than differences in efficacy of the treatment regimens. The more definitive approach to therapy evaluation requires a randomized clinical trial that helps to ensure comparability of the patient characteristics and the disease characteristics of the two treatment groups.

Definition of Study Starting Point. The starting time for determining survival of patients depends on the purpose of the study. For example, the starting time for studying the natural history of a particular cancer might be defined in reference to the appearance of the first symptom. Various reference dates are commonly used as starting times for evaluating the effects of therapy. These include (1) date of diagnosis, (2) date of first visit to physician or clinic, (3) date of hospital admission, (4) date of treatment initiation, date of randomization in a clinical trial evaluating treatment efficacy, and (5) others. The specific reference date used should be clearly specified in every report.

Vital Status. At any given time, the vital status of each patient is defined as alive, dead, or unknown (i.e., lost to follow-up). The endpoint of each patient's participation in the study is (1) a specified *terminal event* such as death, (2) survival to the completion of the study, or (3) loss to follow-up. In each case, the observed follow-up time is the time from the starting point to the terminal event, to the end of the study, or to the date of last observation. This observed follow-up may be further described in terms of patient status at the endpoint, such as the following:
- Alive; tumour-free; no recurrence
- Alive; tumour-free; after recurrence
- Alive with persistent, recurrent, or metastatic disease
- Alive with primary tumour
- Dead; tumour-free
- Dead; with cancer (primary, recurrent, or metastatic disease)
- Dead; postoperative
- Unknown; lost to follow-up

Completeness of the follow-up is crucial in any study of survival, because even a small number of patients lost to follow-up may lead to inaccurate or biased results. The maximum possible effect of bias from patients lost to follow-up may be ascertained by calculating a maximum survival rate, assuming that all lost patients lived to the end of the study. A minimum survival rate may be calculated by assuming that all patients lost to follow-up died at the time they were lost.

Time Intervals. The total survival time is often divided into intervals in units of weeks, months, or years. The survival curve for these intervals provides a description of the population under study with respect to the dynamics of survival over a specified time. The time interval used should be selected with regard to the natural history of the disease under consideration. In diseases with a long natural history, the duration of study could be 5–20 years, and survival intervals of 6–12 months will provide a meaningful description of the survival dynamics. If the population being studied has a very poor prognosis (e.g., patients with carcinoma of the esophagus or pancreas), the total duration of study may be 2–3 years, and the survival intervals may be described in terms of 1–3 months. In interpreting survival rates, one must also take into account the number of individuals entering a survival interval.

Summary
This chapter has reviewed the rudiments of survival analysis as it is often applied

to cancer registry data and to the analysis of data from clinical trials. Complex analysis of data and exploration of research hypotheses demand greater knowledge and expertise than could be conveyed herein. Survival analysis is now performed automatically in many different registry data management and statistical analysis programs available for use on personal computers. Persons with access to these programs are encouraged to explore the different analysis features available to demonstrate for themselves the insight on cancer registry data that survival analysis can provide and to understand the limitations of these analyses and how their validity is affected by the characteristics of the patient cohorts and the quality and completeness of data.

References

1. Cox DR, Oakes D. Analysis of survival data. London: Chapman and Hall; 1984.
2. Fleming TR, Harriton DP. Counting processes and survival analysis, New York; Wiley; 1991
3. Kalbfleisch JD, Prentice RL. The statistical analysis of failure time data. 2nd ed. New York Wiley; 2002
4. Klein JP, Moeschberger ML. Survival analysis: techniques for censored and truncated data. New York: Springer; 1997.
5. Kleinbaum DG. Survival analysis: a self-learning text. New York: Springer; 1996.
6. Lee ET. Statistical methods for survival data analysis. New York: Wiley; 1992
7. Mantel N. Evaluation of survival data and two new rank order statistics arising in its consideration. *Cancer Chemother Rep*. 1966; 50: 163-70.
8. Berkson J, Gage RP. Calculation of survival rates for cancer. *Proc Staff Meet Mayo Clin* 1950;25:270-86.
9. Kaplan EL., Meier P. Nonparametric estimation from incomplete observations. *J Am Stat Assoc* 1958;53:457-81.
10. Ries LAG, Eisner MP, Kosary CL., et al., editors. SEER cancer statistics review, 1973-1997: tables and graphs, National Cancer Institute. Bethesda, MD: National Institutes of Health, NIH Pub. No. 00-2789; 2000.
11. Gooley TA, Leisenring W, Crowley JC, Storer BE. Estimation of failure probabilities in the presence of competing risks; new representations of old estimators. *Stat Med* 1999;18:695-706.
12. Ederer F, Axtell LM, Cutler SJ. The relative survival rate: a statistical methodology. *Natl Cancer Inst Monogr* 1961; 6:101-21.
13. Cox DR. Regression models and life tables. *J R Stat Soc B* 1972;34:187-220.

Acknowledgment: *Used with the permission of the Union for International Cancer Control (UICC), Geneva, Switzerland. The original source for this material is in Brierley JB, Gospodarowicz MK, Wittekind C, eds. UICC TNM Classification of Malignant Tumours, 8th edition (2017), published by John Wiley & Sons, Ltd, www.wiley.com.*

2

The Principles of the TNM System

The practice of classifying cancer cases into groups according to anatomical extent, termed 'stage', arose from the observation that survival rates were higher for cases in which the disease was localized than for those in which the disease had extended beyond the organ of origin. The stage of disease at the time of diagnosis is a reflection not only of the rate of growth and extension of the neoplasm but also the type of tumour and the tumour–host relationship.

It is important to record accurate information on the anatomical extent of the disease for each site at the time of diagnosis, to meet the following objectives:

1. to aid the clinician in the planning of treatment
2. to give some indication of prognosis for survival
3. to assist in evaluation of the results of treatment
4. to facilitate the exchange of information between treatment centres
5. to contribute to the continuing investigation of human cancer
6. to support cancer control activities.

Cancer staging is essential to patient care, research, and cancer control. Cancer control activities include direct patient care-related activities, the development and implementation of clinical practice guidelines, and centralized activities such as recording disease extent in cancer registries for surveillance purposes and planning cancer systems. Recording of stage is essential for the evaluation of outcomes of clinical practice and cancer programmes. However, in order to evaluate the long-term outcomes of populations, it is important for the classification to remain stable. There is therefore a conflict between a classification that is updated to include the most current forms of medical knowledge while also maintaining a classification that facilitates longitudinal studies. The UICC TNM Project aims to address both needs.

International agreement on the classification of cancer by extent of disease provides a method of conveying disease extent to others without ambiguity.

There are many axes of tumour classification: for example, the anatomical site and the clinical and pathological extent of disease, the duration of symptoms or signs, the gender and age of the patient, and the histological type and grade of the tumour. All of these have an influence on the outcome of the disease. Classification by anatomical extent of disease is the one with which the TNM system primarily deals.

The clinician's immediate task when meeting a patient with a new diagnosis of cancer is to make a judgment as to prognosis and a decision as to the most effective course of treatment. This judgment and this decision require, among other things, an objective assessment of the anatomical extent of the disease.

To meet the stated objectives a system of classification is needed:

1. that is applicable to all sites regardless of treatment; and
2. that may be supplemented later by further information that becomes available from histopathology and/or surgery.

The TNM system meets these requirements.

The General Rules of the TNM System[a,b]

The TNM system for describing the anatomical extent of disease is based on the assessment of three components:

T – the extent of the primary tumour
N – the absence or presence and extent of regional lymph node metastasis
M – the absence or presence of distant metastasis.

The addition of numbers to these three components indicates the extent of the malignant disease, thus:

T0, T1, T2, T3, T4, N0, N1, N2, N3, M0, M1

In effect, the system is a 'shorthand notation' for describing the extent of a particular malignant tumour.

The general rules applicable to all sites are as follows:

1. All cases should be confirmed microscopically. Any cases not so proved must be reported separately.
2. Two classifications are described for each site, namely:
   a) **Clinical classification:** the pretreatment clinical classification designated **TNM** (or cTNM) is essential to select and evaluate therapy. This is based on evidence acquired before treatment. Such evidence is gathered from physical examination, imaging, endoscopy, biopsy, surgical exploration, and other relevant examinations.

b) **Pathological classification:** the postsurgical histopathological classification, designated **pTNM**, is used to guide adjuvant therapy and provides additional data to estimate prognosis and end results. This is based on evidence acquired before treatment, supplemented or modified by additional evidence acquired from surgery and from pathological examination. The pathological assessment of the primary tumour (pT) entails a resection of the primary tumour or biopsy adequate to evaluate the highest pT category. The pathological assessment of the regional lymph nodes (pN) entails removal of the lymph nodes adequate to validate the absence of regional lymph node metastasis (pN0) or sufficient to evaluate the highest pN category. An excisional biopsy of a lymph node without pathological assessment of the primary is insufficient to fully evaluate the pN category and is a clinical classification. The pathological assessment of distant metastasis (pM) entails microscopic examination of metastatic deposit.

3. After assigning T, N, and M and/or pT, pN, and pM categories, these may be grouped into stages.The TNM classification and stages, are established at diagnosis and must remain unchanged in the medical records. Only for cancer surveillance purposes, clinical and pathological data may be combined when only partial information is available either in the pathological classification or the clinical classification.

4. If there is doubt concerning the correct T, N, or M category to which a particular case should be allotted, then the lower (i.e., less advanced) category should be chosen. This will also be reflected in the stage.

5. In the case of multiple primary tumours in one organ, the tumour with the highest T category should be classified and the multiplicity or the number of tumours should be indicated in parenthesis, e.g., T2(m) or T2(5). In simultaneous bilateral primary cancers of paired organs, each tumour should be classified independently. In tumours of the liver, ovary and fallopian tube, multiplicity is a criterion of T classification, and in tumours of the lung multiplicity may be a criterion of the M classification.

6. Definitions of the TNM categories and stage may be telescoped or expanded for clinical or research purposes as long as the basic definitions recommended are not changed. For instance, any T, N, or M can be divided into subgroups.

Notes

[a] For more details on classification the reader is referred to the TNM Supplement.
[b] An educational module is available on the UICC website www.uicc.org.

Anatomical Regions and Sites

The sites in this classification are listed by code number of the International

Classification of Diseases for Oncology.[1] Each region or site is described under the following headings:

- Rules for classification with the procedures for assessing the T, N, and M categories
- Anatomical sites, and subsites if appropriate
- Definition of the regional lymph nodes
- TNM Clinical classification
- pTNM Pathological classification
- G Histopathological grading if different from that described in the Histopathological Grading section provided further in this chapter
- Stage and prognostic groups
- Prognostic factors grid

TNM Clinical Classification

The following general definitions are used throughout:

T – Primary Tumour

TX   Primary tumour cannot be assessed
T0   No evidence of primary tumour
Tis   Carcinoma in situ
T1–T4   Increasing size and/or local extent of the primary tumour

N – Regional Lymph Nodes

NX   Regional lymph nodes cannot be assessed
N0   No regional lymph node metastasis
N1–N3   Increasing involvement of regional lymph nodes

M – Distant Metastasis*

M0   No distant metastasis
M1   Distant metastasis

Note

*The MX category is considered to be inappropriate as clinical assessment of metastasis can be based on physical examination alone. (The use of MX may result in exclusion from staging.)

The category M1 may be further specified according to the following notation:

Pulmonary   PUL (C34)
Bone marrow   MAR (C42.1)
Osseous   OSS (C40, 41)
Pleura   PLE (C38.4)

Hepatic   HEP (C22)
Peritoneum   PER (C48.1,2)
Brain   BRA (C71)
Adrenals   ADR (C74)
Lymph nodes   LYM (C77)
Skin   SKI (C44)
Others   OTH

Subdivisions of TNM

Subdivisions of some main categories are available for those who need greater specificity (e.g., T1a, T1b or N2a, N2b).

pTNM Pathological Classification

The following general definitions are used throughout:

pT – Primary Tumour

pTX   Primary tumour cannot be assessed histologically
pT0   No histological evidence of primary tumour
pTis   Carcinoma in situ
pT1–4 Increasing size and/or local extent of the primary tumour histologically

pN – Regional Lymph Nodes

pNX   Regional lymph nodes cannot be assessed histologically
pN0   No regional lymph node metastasis histologically
pN1–3 Increasing involvement of regional lymph nodes histologically

Notes

- Direct extension of the primary tumour into lymph nodes is classified as lymph node metastasis.
- Tumour deposits (satellites), i.e., macro- or microscopic nests or nodules, in the lymph drainage area of a primary carcinoma without histological evidence of residual lymph node in the nodule, may represent discontinuous spread, venous invasion (V1/2) or a totally replaced lymph node. If a nodule is considered by the pathologist to be a totally replaced lymph node (generally having a smooth contour), it should be recorded as a positive lymph node, and each such nodule should be counted separately as a lymph node in the final pN determination.
- Metastasis in any lymph node other than regional is classified as a distant metastasis.
- When size is a criterion for pN classification, measurement is made of the metastasis, not of the entire lymph node. The measurement should be that of the largest dimension of the tumour.

- Cases with micrometastasis only, i.e., no metastasis larger than 0.2 cm, can be identified by the addition of '(mi)', e.g., pN1(mi).

Sentinel Lymph Node

The sentinel lymph node is the first lymph node to receive lymphatic drainage from a primary tumour. If it contains metastatic tumour this indicates that other lymph nodes may contain tumour. If it does not contain metastatic tumour, other lymph nodes are not likely to contain tumour. Occasionally, there is more than one sentinel lymph node.

The following designations are applicable when sentinel lymph node assessment is attempted:

(p)NX(sn) Sentinel lymph node could not be assessed
(p)N0(sn) No sentinel lymph node metastasis
(p)N1(sn) Sentinel lymph node metastasis

Isolated Tumour Cells

Isolated tumour cells (ITC) are single tumour cells or small clusters of cells not more than 0.2 mm in greatest extent that can be detected by routine H and E stains or immunohistochemistry. An additional criterion has been proposed in breast cancer to include a cluster of fewer than 200 cells in a single histological cross-section. Others have proposed for other tumour sites that a cluster should have 20 cells or fewer; definitions of ITC may vary by tumour site. ITCs do not typically show evidence of metastatic activity (e.g., proliferation or stromal reaction) or penetration of vascular or lymphatic sinus walls. Cases with ITC in lymph nodes or at distant sites should be classified as N0 or M0, respectively. The same applies to cases with findings suggestive of tumour cells or their components by non-morphological techniques such as flow cytometry or DNA analysis. The exceptions are in malignant melanoma of the skin and Merkel cell carcinoma, wherein ITC in a lymph node are classified as N1. These cases should be analysed separately.[2] Their classification is as follows.

(p)N0   No regional lymph node metastasis histologically, no examination for isolated tumour cells (ITC)
(p)N0(i–)   No regional lymph node metastasis histologically, negative morphological findings for ITC
(p)N0(i+)   No regional lymph node metastasis histologically, positive morphological findings for ITC
(p)N0(mol–) No regional lymph node metastasis histologically, negative non-morphological findings for ITC
(p)N0(mol+) No regional lymph node metastasis histologically, positive non-morphological findings for ITC

Cases with or examined for isolated tumour cells (ITC) in sentinel lymph nodes can be classified as follows:

(p)N0(i–)(sn)	No sentinel lymph node metastasis histologically, negative morphological findings for ITC
(p)N0(i+)(sn)	No sentinel lymph node metastasis histologically, positive morphological findings for ITC
(p)N0(mol–)(sn)	No sentinel lymph node metastasis histologically, negative non-morphological findings for ITC
(p)N0 (mol+)(sn)	No sentinel lymph node metastasis histologically, positive non-morphological findings for ITC

pM – Distant Metastasis*

pM1   Distant metastasis microscopically confirmed

Note

*pM0 and pMX are not valid categories.

The category pM1 may be further specified in the same way as M1 (see TNM Clinical Classification section provided earlier in this chapter).

Isolated tumour cells found in bone marrow with morphological techniques are classified according to the scheme for N, e.g., M0(i+). For non-morphological findings 'mol' is used in addition to M0, e.g., M0 (mol+).

Histopathological Grading

In most sites, further information regarding the primary tumour may be recorded under the following heading:

G – Histopathological Grading

GX   Grade of differentiation cannot be assessed
G1   Well differentiated
G2   Moderately differentiated
G3   Poorly differentiated
G4   Undifferentiated

Notes

- Grades 3 and 4 can be combined in some circumstances as 'G3-4, poorly differentiated or undifferentiated'.
- Special systems of grading are recommended for tumours of breast, corpus uteri, and prostate.

Additional Descriptors

For identification of special cases in the TNM or pTNM classification, the m, y, r, and a symbols may be used. Although they do not affect the stage grouping, they indicate cases needing separate analysis.

m Symbol. The suffix m, in parentheses, is used to indicate the presence of multiple primary tumours at a single site. See TNM rule no. 5.

y Symbol. In those cases in which classification is performed during or following multimodality therapy, the cTNM or pTNM category is identified by a y prefix. The ycTNM or ypTNM categorizes the extent of tumour actually present at the time of that examination. The y categorization is not an estimate of the extent of tumour prior to multimodality therapy.

r Symbol. Recurrent tumours, when classified after a disease-free interval, are identified by the prefix r.

a Symbol. The prefix a indicates that classification is first determined at autopsy.

Optional Descriptors
L – Lymphatic Invasion

LX   Lymphatic invasion cannot be assessed
L0   No lymphatic invasion
L1   Lymphatic invasion

V – Venous Invasion

VX   Venous invasion cannot be assessed
V0   No venous invasion
V1   Microscopic venous invasion
V2   Macroscopic venous invasion

Note

Macroscopic involvement of the wall of veins (with no tumour within the veins) is classified as V2.

Pn – Perineural Invasion

PnX   Perineural invasion cannot be assessed
Pn0   No perineural invasion
Pn1   Perineural invasion

Residual Tumour (R) Classification*

The absence or presence of residual tumour after treatment is described by the symbol R. More details can be found in the TNM Supplement (see Preface, Reference 3).

TNM and pTNM describe the anatomical extent of cancer in general without considering treatment. They can be supplemented by the R classification, which deals with tumour status after treatment. It reflects the effects of therapy, influences further therapeutic procedures, and is a strong predictor of prognosis.

The definitions of the R categories are:

RX   Presence of residual tumour cannot be assessed
R0   No residual tumour
R1   Microscopic residual tumour
R2   Macroscopic residual tumour.

Note

*Some consider the R classification to apply only to the primary tumour and its local or regional extent. Others have applied it more broadly to include distant metastasis. The specific usage should be indicated when the R is used.

Stage and Prognostic Groups

The TNM system is used to describe and record the anatomical extent of disease. For purposes of tabulation and analysis it is useful to condense these categories into groups. For consistency, in the TNM system, carcinoma in situ is categorized stage 0; in general, tumours localized to the organ of origin as stages I and II, locally extensive spread, particularly to regional lymph nodes as stage III, and those with distant metastasis as stage IV. The stage adopted is such as to ensure, as far as possible, that each group is more or less homogeneous in respect of survival, and that the survival rates of these groups for each cancer site are distinctive.

For pathological stages, if sufficient tissue has been removed for pathological examination to evaluate the highest T and N categories, M1 may be either clinical (cM1) or pathological (pM1). However, if only a distant metastasis has had microscopic confirmation, the classification is pathological (pM1) and the stage is pathological.

Although the anatomical extent of disease, as categorized by TNM, is a very powerful prognostic indicator in cancer, it is recognized that many factors have a significant impact on predicting outcomes. This has resulted in different stage groups. In thyroid cancer there are different stage definitions for different histologies and, new to this edition, in oropharyngeal cancer HPV-related cancer is staged differently from non-HPV-related cancer. Some factors have been combined with

TNM in the development of stage groupings; for instance, for different histologies (thyroid), different major prognostic factor groups (age in thyroid), and by aetiology (HPV-related oropharyngeal cancer). In this edition the term **stage** has been used as defining the anatomical extent of disease while **prognostic group** for classifications that incorporate other prognostic factors. Historically, age in differentiated thyroid cancer and grade in soft tissue sarcoma are combined with anatomical extent of disease to determine stage, and stage is retained rather than prognostic group in these two sites.

Prognostic Factors Classification

Prognostic factors can be classified as those pertaining to:

- **Anatomic extent of disease:** describes the extent of disease in the patient at the time of diagnosis. Classically, this is TNM but may also include tumour markers that reflect tumour burden, for instance prostate-specific antigen (PSA) in prostate carcinoma or carcinoembryonic antigen (CEA) in colorectal carcinoma.
- **Tumour profile:** this includes pathological (i.e., grade) and molecular features of a tumour, and gene expression patterns that reflect behaviour. These can be:
  - predictive factors
  - prognostic factors
  - companion diagnostic marker
- **Patient profile:** this includes terms related to the host of the cancer. These can be demographic factors, such as age and gender, or acquired, such as immunodeficiency and performance status.
- **Environment:** this may include treatment-related and education (expertise, access, ageism, and healthcare delivery) and quality of management.

When describing prognostic factors it is important to state what outcome the factors are prognostic for, and at what point in the patient trajectory. Anatomical extent of disease as described by TNM stage defines prognosis for survival.

In the second edition of the *UICC Prognostic Factors in Cancer* for each tumour site, grids were developed that identified prognostic factors for survival at time of diagnosis and whether they were considered to be essential, additional, or new and promising.[3] The grids were updated for the third edition[4] and have been further updated and incorporated into the ninth edition of the *UICC Manual of Clinical Oncology*.[5] Essential factors are those that are required in addition to anatomical extent of disease to determine treatment as identified by published clinical practice guidelines. The table is a generic example of the prognostic factors summary grid. The grids from the ninth edition of the *UICC Manual of Clinical Oncology* are reproduced in this eighth edition. Grids are not available for some of the less common tumours.

Examples of the UICC prognostic factors summary 'grid'

Prognostic Factors	Tumour Related	Host Related	Environment Related
Essential*	Anatomical disease extent Histological type	Age	Availability of access to radiotherapy
Additional	Tumour bulk Tumour marker level Programmed death 1 (PD-1) receptor and its ligands (PD-L1)	Race Gender Cardiac function	Expertise of a treatment at the specific level (e.g., surgery or radiotherapy)
New and promising	Epidermal growth factor receptor Gene expression patterns	Germline p53	Access to information

*The origin of essential factors as imperatives for treatment decisions are from known and available clinical practice guidelines.

Essential TNM

Information on anatomical extent of disease at presentation or stage is central to cancer surveillance to determine cancer burden as it provides additional valuable information to incidence and mortality data.[6] However, cancer registries in low and middle income countries frequently have insufficient information to determine complete TNM data, either because of inability to perform necessary investigations or because of lack of recording of information. In view of this, the UICC TNM Project has with the International Agency for Research in Cancer and the National Cancer Institute developed a new classification system 'Essential TNM' that can be used to collect stage data when complete information is not available. To date, Essential TNM schemas have been developed for breast, cervix, colon, and prostate cancer, and are presented in this edition and available for download at www.uicc.org.

Paediatric Tumours

Since the fourth edition, the *UICC TNM Classification of Malignant Tumours* has not incorporated any classifications of paediatric tumours. This decision has stemmed from the lack of an international standard staging system for many paediatric tumours. To enable stage data collection by population-based cancer registries there needs to be agreement on cancer staging. Recognition of this led to a consensus meeting held in 2014 and resulted in the publication of recommendations on the staging of paediatric malignancies for the purposes of population surveillance.[7] The classifications published are not intended to replace the classifications used by the clinician when treating an individual patient but instead to facilitate the collection of stage by population-based cancer registries.

Related Classifications

Since 1958, WHO has been involved in a programme aimed at providing internationally acceptable criteria for the histological diagnosis of tumours. This has resulted in the *International Histological Classification of Tumours,* which contains, in an illustrated multivolume series, definitions of tumour types and a proposed nomenclature. A new series, *WHO Classification of Tumours–Pathology and Genetics of Tumours,* continues this effort. (Information on these publications is at www.iarc.fr).

The *WHO International Classification of Diseases for Oncology (ICD-O-3)*[1] is a coding system for neoplasms by topography and morphology and for indicating behaviour (e.g., malignant, benign). This coded nomenclature is identical in the morphology field for neoplasms to the Systematized Nomenclature of Medicine (SNOMED).[8]

In the interest of promoting national and international collaboration in cancer research and specifically of facilitating cooperation in clinical investigations, it is recommended that the WHO *Classification of Tumours* be used for classification and definition of tumour types and that the ICD-O-3 code be used for storage and retrieval of data.

References

1. Fritz A, Percy C, Jack A, Shanmugaratnam K, Sobin L, Parkin DM, Whelan S, eds. *WHO International Classification of Diseases for Oncology ICD-O,* 3rd edn. Geneva: WHO, 2000.
2. Hermanek P, Hutter RVP, Sobin LH, Wittekind Ch. Classification of isolated tumour cells and micrometastasis. *Cancer* 1999; 86: 2668–2673.
3. International Union Against Cancer (UICC) Gospodarowicz MK, Henson DE, Hutter RVP, et al., eds. *Prognostic Factors in Cancer,* 2nd edn. New York: Wiley, 2001.
4. International Union Against Cancer (UICC) Gospodarowicz MK, O'Sullivan B, Sobin LH, eds. *Prognostic Factors in Cancer,* 3rd edn. New York: Wiley, 2006.
5. O'Sullivan B, Brierley J, D'Cruz A, Fey M, Pollock R, Vermorken J, Huang S. *Manual of Clinical Oncology,* 9th edn. Oxford: Wiley-Blackwell, 2015.
6. The World Health Organization. *Cancer Control Knowledge into Action, Guide for Effective Programs.* Available at: www.who.int/cancer/modules/en/(accessed Aug. 2016).
7. Gupta S, Aitken J, Bartels U, et al. Paediatric cancer stage in population-based cancer registries: the Toronto consensus principles and guidelines. *Lancet Oncol* 2016; 17: e163–172.
8. SNOMED International: *The Systematized Nomenclature of Human and Veterinary Medicine.* Northfield, Ill: College of American Pathologists. Available at: www.cap.org (accessed Aug. 2016).

PART II

LUNG CANCER

Executive Editor's Note: *Prof. Peter Goldstraw's involvement with the IASLC Staging Project spanned 13 years at the time of publication (2009) of the first edition of the IASLC* Staging Manual in Thoracic Oncology *of which he was Executive Editor. During that time, he gained some insight into the origins and development of the TNM classification for lung cancer, the important part played by a few far-sighted and industrious individuals and the ralationship between the two bodies that now administer the system worldwide, the Union for International Cancer Control (UICC) and the American Joint Committee on Cancer (AJCC). Through the good offices of Drs. Leslie Sobin, Brian O'Sullivan, and Thierry le Chevalier, Prof. Goldstraw had access to the archives of the UICC and of the Institute Gustave Roussy. The archives were degrading and many important documents were already lost. This chapter will allow the reader to understand the motives that led to the establishment of the IASLC Staging Project and to appreciate why this has proven to be such a milestone in the development of TNM, not only in lung cancer, but also in malignant pleural mesothelioma and thymic epithelial tumours, for which it provided a template to accomplish similar initiatives.*

3

The History of TNM Staging in Lung Cancer

Peter Goldstraw

Efforts to develop an international language for the classification of cancer by describing the anatomical extent of disease started at the beginning of the 20th century.[1] During the first half of that century a number of organizations attempted to develop such systems and there were attempts to achieve an international consensus. From 1929 the lead was taken by the Radiological Sub-Commission of the Cancer Commission of the League of Nations Health Organization. They developed rules and definitions, created a classification by the anatomical extent of disease, identified the data elements required for the assessment of the results of treatment and went on to produce an Atlas, in 3 languages, showing the classification of cancer by stage. Although primarily concerned with carcinoma of the cervix these principles were widely accepted by other organizations. In 1950 three other organizations established committees to focus on this aspect of cancer: the World Health Organization Expert Committee on Health Statistics established its sub-committee on the Registration of Cases of Cancer as well as their Statistical Presentation, the 6th International Congress of Radiology created the International Commission on Stage-Grouping in Cancer and Presentation of the Results of Cancer (ICPR) and the Union Internationale Contre le Cancer (UICC) founded in Paris in 1934, now the International Union Against Cancer, established a Committee on Tumour Nomenclature and Statistics (CTNS).

During this period Professor Pierre Denoix (Figure 3.1), a surgeon at the Institut Gustave-Roussy in Paris, developed his system for the classification of malignant tumours, based upon "TNM," publishing a series of articles between 1943 and 1952[2]. He presented his "Uniform Technique for Clinical Classification by the TNM System" at the 7th International Congress of Radiology in 1953, and thereafter the ICPR adopted TNM as the basis of its classification for cancer of the larynx and breast. The next year the UICC replaced the CTNS with a special Committee on Clinical Stage Classification and Applied Statistics (CCSCAS) under the

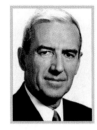

Figure 3.1. Dr. Pierre Denoix, 1912–1990. Surgical oncologist at the Institut Gustave-Roussy, Paris, Director of the Institut Gustave-Roussy 1956–1982. Chairman of the UICC Committee on Clinical Stage Classification and Applied Statistics, 1954–1966. President of the UICC 1973–1978. Commander of the Legion of Honour.

chairmanship of Professor Denoix. For the next 4 years this committee refined the general principles of TNM and undertook extensive international consultation on its proposals. The UICC then undertook a program to publish brochures or "fascicles" in which TNM classifications were proposed for cancer in different organ sites. In all, between 1960 and 1967, nine brochures were produced covering 23 sites, lung being included in a brochure published in 1966. The intention was to review the proposals for each site after a 5 year period of "field trials." In 1966 the UICC replaced the CCSCAS with a Committee of TNM Classification under the chairmanship of Mr. Michael Harmer. At this time the UICC was using both the French and Anglophone versions of its title, but gradually came to prefer the Anglicized form, while retaining the French abbreviation.

In 1968 the proposals contained in the brochures were brought together in the UICC "TNM Classification of Malignant Tumours,"[3] lung cancer being included under the section on "other sites." The T descriptors, in this first classification for lung cancer, included T0 for cases in which one could find no evidence of the primary tumour, T1 for tumours confined to a segmental bronchus or to a segment of one lobe, T2 in which tumour was confined to a lobar bronchus or one lobe, T3 in which tumour was involving the main bronchus or more than one lobe, and T4 for tumours extending beyond the lung. The N descriptors were NX, N0 and N1, in which there was "enlargement" of "intrathoracic" lymph nodes on "clinical, radiological or endoscopic evidence." These intrathoracic lymph nodes were further divided into "hilar" or "peripheral" nodes, but as yet, there was no mention of nodes in the mediastinum. The M1 category was sub-divided into M1a, in which there was a pleural effusion with malignant cells, M1b cases with "palpable" cervical nodes and M1c for cases in which there were other distant metastases. Stage groupings were not proposed at this time and the classification was restricted to recording the anatomical extent of disease following clinical evaluation, subsequently designated as cTNM.

The American Joint Committee for Cancer Staging and End Results Reporting (AJC) was created in 1959, with representatives of the American College of Radiology, the American College of Surgeons, the College of American Pathologists, the American College of Physicians, the American Cancer Society and the National Cancer Institute. In 1980 it was renamed as the American Joint Committee on

Cancer (AJCC). The AJC developed a separate and distinctive process from that of the UICC, employing "Task Forces" to gather data on specific cancer sites and to use this data to inform its proposals. The emergence of this new organization refocused American participation away from the UICC and resulted in the possibility that these two organizations could make different, and possibly conflicting, recommendations to the cancer community. In 1968 there followed a series of meetings between the AJC and UICC and finally a "rapprochement" was reached, ensuring that neither would publish further recommendations without consultation with the other. In 1969 this agreement was extended to include "as far as practicable, other National TNM Committees and International non-governmental professional organizations."

In 1973 Drs. Mountain, Carr, and Anderson reported the results of a study, undertaken under the auspices of the Task Force on Lung Cancer of the AJC, to develop "A Clinical Staging System for Lung Cancer."[4] Their proposals were derived from a data base of 2,155 cases of lung cancer, of which 1,712 were cases of non-small cell lung cancer (NSCLC), diagnosed at least 4 years before analysis. Practically all of the T descriptors in use today were introduced in that report, including the use of a 3 cm cut-off point for size, the impact on T category of invasion of the visceral and parietal pleura, the chest wall, diaphragm and mediastinum, the bronchoscopic criteria of T category and those based upon the extent of atelectasis or obstructive pneumonitis. The T categories proposed by the UICC were reduced with the loss of the T4 category, but an N2 category was added to address the issue of mediastinal node involvement. Malignant pleural effusion was reclassified from M1 to become a T3 descriptor. For the first time, the concept of stage groups was introduced, incorporating TNM subsets with similar prognoses "in a manner intended to minimize intragroup variability in survival and to create the greatest prognostic differences between stage groups." There were 18 possible permutations of the T, N, and M categories, grouped into stages I, II, and III. Four of the possible TNM sets had too few cases for analysis and 7 others contained less than 100 cases, 1 as few as 24. Stage I included T1 N0 M0, T2 N0 M0, and T1 N1 M0 subsets; Stage II accommodated T2 N1 M0 cases; and the other 14 TNM subsets all fell within Stage III. Graphs showed distinct differences in 5-year survival between each of the T, N, and M categories and the three stage groupings. A table showed different survival at 12 and 18 months for those TNM sets for which data were available, but no validation was presented for any of the individual descriptors. These proposals, although somewhat flawed in retrospect, represented the first attempt at data-driven revisions to the TNM classification of lung cancer. They were incorporated into the 2nd edition of the UICC TNM Classification of Malignant Tumours published in 1975[5] and the 1st edition of the Manual for Staging of Cancer published by the AJC in 1977.[6]

The 3rd edition of the UICC manual, published in 1978[7] and enlarged and revised in 1982, was approved by National TNM committees in Canada, Germany, and Japan and the ICPR. In this edition, Stage I was further divided into Ia and Ib (N.B. at that time stage sub-groups were lower case) and stage IV was established for M1 disease. For the first time a separate classification was established to record the post-surgical histopathologic extent of disease (pTNM), and additional descriptors were introduced of "y" to identify classification performed during or following initial multimodality therapy and "r" for classification of recurrent tumours after a disease-free interval, and the optional use of the "C" factor was allowed to reflect the validity of classification according to the diagnostic methods employed. The Americans, however, were still using the previous classification which was published, without change, as the 2nd edition of their manual in 1983,[8] now under the auspices of the AJCC.

In 1986 Dr. Mountain (Figure 3.2) published "A new International Staging System for Lung Cancer"[9] based upon his own database which, at that time, contained 3,753 cases of lung cancer with a minimum follow-up of 2 years. His proposals were widely discussed at meetings held in 1985 between the AJCC, the UICC, and cancer committees from Germany and Japan, and when accepted, once more brought into line the classification of lung cancer in 4th edition of the UICC manual, published in 1987[10] and the 3rd edition of the American manual published in 1988.[11] The changes that now came into force included the classification of superficial tumours in which invasion was limited to the bronchial wall as T1 irrespective of location, the recommendation that the occasional pleural effusion that was cytologically negative could be ignored in defining the T category, the re-emergence of the T4 category and the creation of an N3 category. The existing T3 descriptors were split between the T3 category and the new T4 category on the basis that the former would retain those tumours that were "candidates for complete resection" while the latter category would contain tumours which were considered to be "inoperable." The previous descriptor of "mediastinal invasion" was split into its component parts, with invasion of the mediastinal pleura or pericardium remaining T3 descriptors while invasion of the great vessels, heart, trachea, oesophagus, carina and vertebral bodies became T4 descriptors, along with the presence of a pleural effusion. The situation was confused by the additional definitions of the T3 and T4 categories given in the text. Those tumours with "limited, circumscribed extrapulmonary extension" were to be retained within the T3 category while those with "extensive extrapulmonary

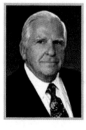

Figure 3.2. Dr. Clifton Fletcher Mountain, 1924–2007. Thoracic Surgeon, Chief of Thoracic Surgery, Chair of Surgical Department, MD Anderson 1960–1996. Founding member of the IASLC 1973, and President 1977.

extension" now fell into the new T4 category. These conflicting definitions caused some confusion. Were tumours invading such structures as the pericardium still classified as T3 even if there was extensive invasion and they were considered inoperable? Or, in such circumstances did they become T4? If invasion of the oesophagus was limited to a circumscribed area of the muscular wall and could be resected completely at surgery should these cases be classified as T3 or T4? Metastases to the ipsilateral mediastinal nodes and subcarinal nodes remained within the N2 category, and a new N3 category was added to accommodate metastases to the contralateral mediastinal nodes, contralateral hilum or ipsilateral and contralateral supraclavicular or scalene lymph nodes. Additional changes in the new classification involved the moving of T1 N1 M0 cases from stage I to stage II and the division of stage III into IIIA, to accommodate T3 and N2 cases and IIIB, to accommodate the T4 and N3 categories (note, although stage subsets were identified by the use of the lower case in the original article by Dr. Mountain, upper case was now used for the first time in both the UICC and American manuals). The survival of those clinical and pathological TNM subsets that fell within stages I to IIIA and stage IV were shown to differ but no statistical analysis was presented. However, a graph showed statistically significant differences in survival between stage groupings. Once again there was no validation of any of the individual descriptors contained in these recommendations.

The AJCC published its 4th edition of TNM in 1992.[12] There were no changes for lung cancer. However, for the first time pleural mesothelioma was included, as a separate chapter.

At the time of the next revision in 1997 the database of Dr. Mountain had grown to include 5,319 cases, all but 66 being NSCLC. Of these, 4,351 cases had been treated at the M D Anderson Cancer Centre between 1975 and 1988 and documentation on a further 968 cases had been sent there from the National Cancer Institute cooperative Lung Cancer Study Group for confirmation of stage and histology.[13] Tables showed statistically significant differences in survival to 5 years between clinical/evaluative cTNM subsets and pathological/post-surgical pTNM subsets T1 N0 M0 and T2 N0 M0 and these were divided into a new stage IA and stage IB respectively. Similarly T1 N1 M0 cases were placed in a new stage IIA and T2 N1 M0 and T3 N0 M0 cases became stage IIB. The remaining TNM subsets in stages IIIA, IIIB and IV remained unchanged although statistically significant differences were found between some of these subsets. An additional paragraph determined that "the presence of *satellite* tumours within the primary-tumour lobe of the lung should be classified as T4. Intrapulmonary ipsilateral *metastasis* in a distant, that is, nonprimary lobe(s) of the lung, should be classified M1." No data was presented to support these suggestions and the wording used to describe such additional pulmonary nodules was loaded to underline the apparent logic of considering some to be "satellite" lesions and therefore fell into a T category while those in other lobes were a "metastasis" and therefore fell into an M category. These recommendations were accepted by the AJCC and the UICC-TNM Prognostic Factors Project Committee, and were incorporated in to their 5th editions, published 1997.[14,15]

The International Association for the Study of Lung Cancer (IASLC) Lung Cancer Staging Project

At an IASLC sponsored workshop in London in 1996[16] Dr. Mountain presented his proposals for the forthcoming 5th edition of TNM. The Mountain database by this time had enlarged to include 5,319 cases, still relatively small, but this had been accumulated over 20 years, during which time many advances had been made in clinical staging, most importantly the routine application of computed tomography (CT) scanning. This database was mostly populated with surgical cases leading many oncologists unsure as to whether TNM had any relevance in non-surgical cases. The database reflected practice in one part of the world but informed an International classification. The lack of validation in previous editions of the TNM classification led to many of the descriptors being increasingly challenged by data from other sources. Because of these limitations, the delegates at the workshop felt that there was a need to develop a new database to inform future revisions of the TNM classification. It was suggested that the IASLC, as the only global organization dedicated to the study of lung cancer, representing all clinical and research aspects of lung cancer care, had a responsibility to become involved in the revision process. A proposal to this effect was included in the conclusions of the workshop[16] and placed before the board of the IASLC at the 8th World Conference on Lung Cancer held in Dublin in 1997. In December 1998 the board agreed to this proposal and granted pump-priming funds for the project. Meetings were held in London in 1999 and 2000 during which the composition of the committee was developed to ensure speciality and geographical representation and the involvement of stakeholders such as the UICC, the AJCC, the European Lung Cancer Working Group and the joint Japanese lung cancer societies. At the 9th World Conference held in Tokyo in 2000 the committee was joined by colleagues from Cancer Research And Biostatistics (CRAB), a not-for-profit medical statistics and data management organization based in Seattle with extensive experience with multi-centre data collection and analysis. At that meeting sufficient funds were guaranteed from the pharmaceutical industry to allow a major meeting in London in 2001 to which database proprietors were invited to present their data. Over the 2-day workshop data on 80,000 cases was presented from 20 databases across the globe. In was decided to base the budget required to continue this project upon the assumption that 30,000 suitable cases could be recruited and that the length of the project would be the 5-year cycle of revision proposed by the UICC and AJCC at that time. Cases would be solicited from databases world wide, treated by all modalities of care, registered between 1990 and 2000, a period during which there had been relative stability in staging methods. This would ensure a 5-year follow-up by the time of analysis. In collaboration with CRAB the data fields and data dictionary were finalized. Later that year full funding was obtained by the IASLC via a partnership agreement with a pharmaceutical company.

As the UICC and AJCC were aware of the progress of this initiative they decided that no changes should be made to lung cancer classification in the 6th editions of their manuals published in 2002.[17,18]

Meetings of the IASLC staging committee were held on an annual basis utilizing the World Conferences, now held biennially, wherever possible. In May 2003 the UICC and AJCC extended the revision cycle to 7 years and proposed that the 7th edition of the TNM would be published early in 2009. The internal review processes within these two organizations would require that the IASLC proposals be submitted to the UICC in January 2007 and the AJCC in June 2008.

Data collection was discontinued in April 2005 by which time over 100,000 cases had been submitted to the data centre at CRAB. After an initial sift which excluded cases with insufficient data on stage, treatment or follow-up, cases outside the designated study period and cases in which the cell type was unsuited or unknown 81,495 were available for analysis, 68,463 cases of NSCLC and 13,032 cases of small-cell lung cancer (SCLC) (Table 3.1). The geographical distribution of the data sources is illustrated in Figure 3.3 and the spread of treatment modalities is shown in Figure 3.4.

At the 11th World Conference in Barcelona in July 2005 subcommittees were established to develop the proposals for key aspects of the project. Additional subgroups were later added (Table 3.2). It was agreed that the membership of the IASLC, and the wider lung cancer community would be informed of the progress of the work through discussion

Table 3.1. Summary of cases contributed to the IASLC Staging Project.

Total Cases Submitted	100,869
Excluded From Current Analyses	**19,374**
- Outside of 1990-2000 Time Frame	5,467
- Incomplete Survival Data	1,192
- Unknown Histology	2,419
- Incomplete Stage Information	8,075
- Recurrent Cases and Other (e.g. Not known if recurrent vs. newly diagnosed, occult tumors)	1093
- Carcinoids, Sarcomas, other histologies	1,128
Included in Analyses	**81,495**
- SCLC	13,032
- NSCLC	68,463

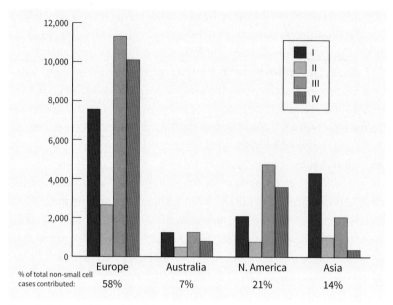

Figure 3.3. Geographical origin of data for IASLC Staging Project.

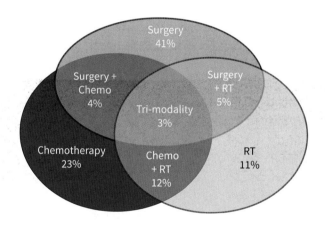

Figure 3.4. Treatment modalities of cases within the IASLC Staging Project.

articles to be published in the *Journal of Thoracic Oncology* (JTO), the official journal of the IASLC.[19]

Intensive validation was crucially important in this project and the lack of it in earlier editions had been a major motive for the development of the project. A validation and methodology sub-committee was therefore established and was intimately involved in the analyses conducted by CRAB and the development of the proposals from each sub-committee.[20] Internal validity was undertaken by ensuring that all of the proposals were supported across different types of databases and in most geographical areas. External validity was assured by testing the new proposals against the SEER data base for the relevant period.

Where the analyses showed descriptors to have a prognosis that differed from the other descriptors in any T or M category, two alternative strategies were considered. First, retain that descriptor in the existing category, identified by alphabetical subscripts. For example, additional pulmonary nodules in the lobe of the primary, considered to be T4 in the 6th edition of TNM, would become T4a, while additional pulmonary nodules in other ipsilateral lobes, designated as M1 in the 6th edition, would become M1a. Second, allow descriptors to move between categories, to a category containing other descriptors with a similar prognosis, e.g. additional pulmonary nodules in the lobe of the primary would move from T4 to T3, and additional pulmonary nodules in other ipsilateral lobes would move from M1 to T4. The first strategy had the advantage of allowing, to a large extent, retrograde compatibility with existing databases. Unfortunately this generated a large number of descriptors (approximately 20) and an impractically large number of TNM subsets (over 180). For this reason backwards compatibility was compromised and strategy ii) was preferred for its clinical use. The resultant T, N, and M categories were incorporated into new TNM subsets and a small number of candidate stage groupings were developed using a recursive partitioning and amalgamation (RPA) algorithm.[21] The analysis grouped cases based on best stage (pathologic if available, otherwise clinical) after determination of best-split points based on overall survival on indicator variables for the newly proposed T/M categories and an ordered variable for N-category, excluding NX cases. This analysis was performed on a ran-

Table 3.2. Membership of the sub-committees of the IASLC Staging Project.

T-Descriptors

Chairperson Ramon Rami-Porta
David Ball
John Crowley
Peter Goldstraw
James Jett
William Travis
Masahiro Tsuboi
Eric Vallieres

N-Descriptors

Chairperson Valerie Rusch
John Crowley
Jung-Gi Im
Peter Goldstraw
Ryosuke Tsuchiya
Johan Vansteenkiste

Prognostic Factors

Chairperson Jean-Paul Sculier
John Crowley
Peter Goldstraw
Thierry Le Chevalier
Jan van Meerbeeck

Small Cell Lung Cancer

Chairperson Frances A. Shepherd
Desmond Carney
John Crowley
Peter Goldstraw
Paul Van Houtte
Pieter E. Postmus

Validation and Methodology

Chairperson Patti Groome
John Crowley
Peter Goldstraw
Catherine Kennedy
Leslie Sobin
Mark Krasnik

M-Descriptors

Chairperson Pieter Postmus
Elizabeth Brambilla
John Crowley
Peter Goldstraw
Ned Patz
Hiroyasu Yokomise

Nodal Chart

Chairperson: Ryosuke Tsuchiya
David Ball
John Crowley
Peter Goldstraw
Edward Patz

domly selected training set comprising two-thirds of the available data that met the requirements for conversion to newly proposed T and M categories (N=17,726), reserving 9,133 cases for later validation. The random selection process was stratified by type of database submission and time period of case entry (1990-1995 vs 1995-2000). The RPA analysis generated a tree-based model for the survival data using log-rank test statistics for recursive partitioning and, for selection of the important groupings, bootstrap re-sampling to correct for the adaptive nature of the splitting algorithm. With an ordered list of groupings from the terminal nodes of the "survival tree" as a guide, several proposed stage groupings were created by combining adjacent groups. Selection of a final stage grouping proposal from among the candidate schemes was based upon its statistical properties in the training set and its relevance to clinical practice, and was arrived at by consensus.

The proposals from the project were submitted to the board of the IASLC in September 2006 and were approved unanimously. The recommendations regarding T, N, and M descriptors and the TNM stage groupings[22-25] were submitted to the UICC in December 2006 and to the AJCC in June 2007. The committee subsequently produced additional proposals: a) confirming and reinforcing the validity of the TNM classification in the clinical staging of SCLC,[26] b) demonstrating the use of TNM for the classification of broncho-pulmonary carcinoid tumours,[27] leading to the inclusion of carcinoid tumours for the first time in the 7th edition of TNM, c) the value of additional, and independent prognostic factors in the clinical and pathological TNM populations,[28,29] d) proposals for an international "IASLC" nodal chart that for the first time reconciled the differences in the Naruke and Mountain/Dresler nodal charts, allowing one chart to be used globally with consequent improvement in data collection and analysis,[30] and e) providing a clear definition of "visceral pleural invasion" a T2a descriptor.[31]

The IASLC Lung Cancer Staging Project has involved a great deal of work, not only from the members of the committee and our colleagues at CRAB but also from those Institutions that generously donated their data so that the project could succeed. The Lung Cancer community has much for which to thank these individuals.

The 7th edition of TNM in lung cancer is unique. It is the first classification to be based upon global data, data on cases treated by all modalities of care, and to have been intensively validated internally and externally. There will be questions raised about existing treatment algorithms.[32] It may be possible to get some data from the re-analysis of published studies but undoubtedly there will be a need for new prospective trials. The limitations inherent in a study that has been based upon retrospective data, notably imbalances and deficiencies in geographical recruitment and the spread of treatment modalities, and others, will be addressed in the next phase of the IASLC Staging Project. The prospective data set has been published[33] and a web-based data collection system is being developed. The project will be expanded to cover the neuroendocrine tumours of the lung, first covered by the WHO classification in 1999,[34,35] and mesothelioma. We hope that colleagues around the world will continue to support and contribute to this initiative, to ensure that the TNM classification is further improved in future editions.

References

1. Sellers TA. The Classification of Malignant Tumours by Anatomical Extent of Disease: The Development of the TNM System. 1980.
2. Denoix PF. The TNM Staging System. *Bull Inst Nat Hyg* (Paris) 1952; 7: 743.
3. UICC. TNM Classification of Malignant Tumours. 1st. 1968. Geneva, UICC.
4. Mountain CF, Carr DT, Anderson WAD. A system for the clinical staging of lung cancer. *Am J Roentgenol Rad Ther Nucl Med* 1974;120: 130-138.
5. UICC. TNM Classification of Malignant Tumours. 2nd. 1975. Geneva, UICC.
6. American Joint Committee on Cancer Staging and End Results Reporting. AJC Cancer Staging Manual. 1st ed. Philadelphia: Lippincott-Raven; 1977.
7. UICC. TNM Classification of Malignant Tumours. 3rd. 1978. Geneva, UICC.
8. American Joint Committee on Cancer. Manual for Staging of Cancer. Beahrs OH, Myers MH, editors. 2nd ed. Philadelphia, J.B. Lippincott Co.; 1983.
9. Mountain CF. A new international staging system for lung cancer. *Chest* 1986;89S:225S-32S.
10. Hermanek P, Sobin LH, UICC. TNM Classification of Malignant Tumours. 4th ed. Berlin, Springer Verlag; 1987.
11. American Joint Committee on Cancer. Manual for Staging of Cancer. Beahrs OH, Henson DE, Hutter RVP, Myers MH, editors. 3rd ed.Philadelphia, J.B. Lippincott Co. ; 1988.
12. American Joint Committee on Cancer. Manual for Staging of Cancer. Beahrs OH, Henson DE, Hutter RVP, Kennedy BJ, editors. 4th ed. Philadelphia, J.B. Lippincott Co.; 1992.
13. Mountain CF. Revisions in the International System for Staging Lung Cancer. Chest 1997; 111: 1710-1717.
14. UICC International Union Against Cancer. TNM Classification of Malignant Tumours. Sobin LH, Wittekind C, editors. 5th ed. New York, Wiley-Liss; 1997.
15. American Joint Committee on Cancer. AJCC Cancer Staging Manual. Fleming ID, Cooper JS, Henson DE, Hutter RVP, Kennedy BJ, Murphy GP et al., editors. 5th ed. Philadelphia, Lipincott Raven; 1997.
16. Goldstraw P. Report on the International workshop on intrathoracic staging. London, October 1996. *Lung Cancer* 1997; 18: 107-111.
17. UICC International Union Against Cancer. TNM Classification of Malignant Tumours. 6th ed. New York: Wiley-Liss; 2002.
18. American Joint Committee on Cancer. AJCC Cancer Staging Manual. 6th ed. New York: Springer; 2002.
19. Goldstraw P, Crowley J, IASLC International Staging Project. The IASLC International Staging Project on Lung Cancer. *J Thorac Oncol* 2006; 1: 281-286.
20. Groome PA, Bolejack V, Crowley JJ, Kennedy C, Krasnik M, Sobin LH, et al. The IASLC Lung Cancer Staging Project: validation of the proposals for revision of the T, N and M descriptors and consequent stage groupings in the forthcoming (seventh) TNM classification for lung cancer. *J Thorac Oncol* 2007; 2: 694-705.
21. Crowley JJ, LeBlanc M, Jacobson J, et al. Some exploratory tools for survival analysis. In: Lin DY, Fleming TR, editors. Proceedings of the First Seattle Symposium in Biostatistics: Survival analysis.. 1st ed. New York: Sprimger; 1997. p. 199-229.
22. Rami-Porta R, Ball D, Crowley JJ, Giroux DJ, Jett JR, Travis WD, et al. The IASLC Lung Cancer Staging Project: proposals for the revision of the T descriptors in the forthcoming (seventh) edition of the TNM classification for lung cancer. *J Thorac Oncol* 2007;2: 593-602.

23. Rusch VR, Crowley JJ, Giroux DJ, Goldstraw P, Im J-G, Tsuboi M, et al. The IASLC Lung Cancer Staging Project: proposals for revision of the N descriptors in the forthcoming (seventh) edition of the TNM classification for lung cancer. *J Thorac Oncol* 2007; 2: 603-612.

24. Postmus PE, Brambilla E, Chansky K, Crowley J, Goldstraw P, Patz EF, et al. The IASLC Lung Cancer Staging Project: proposals for revision of the M descriptors in the forthcoming (seventh) edition of the TNM classification for lung cancer. *J Thorac Oncol* 2007;2: 686-693.

25. Goldstraw P, Crowley JJ, Chansky K, Giroux DJ, Groome PA, Rami-Porta R, et al. The IASLC Lung Cancer Staging Project: proposals for revision of the stage groupings in the forthcoming (seventh) edition of the TNM classification for lung cancer. *J Thorac Oncol* 2007; 2: 706-714.

26. Shepherd FA, Crowley J, Van Houtte P, Postmus PE, Carney D, Chansky K, et al. The IASLC Lung Cancer Staging Project: proposals regarding the clinical staging of small-cell lung cancer in the forthcoming (seventh) edition of the TNM classification for lung cancer. *J Thorac Oncol* 2007; 2: 1067-1077.

27. Travis WD, Giroux DJ, Chansky K, Crowley J, Asamura H, Brambilla E, et al. The IASLC Lung Cancer Staging Project: proposals for the inclusion of bronchopulmonary carcinoid tumours in the forthcoming (seventh) edition of the TNM classification for lung cancer. *J Thorac Oncol* 2008; 3: 1213-1223.

28. Sculier JP, Chansky K, Crowley JJ, van Meerbeeck JV, Goldstraw P. The impact of additional prognostic factors on survival and their relationship with the anatomical extent of disease expressed by the 6th edition of the TNM classification of malignant tumors and the proposals for the 7th edition. *J Thorac Oncol* 2008; 3: 457-466.

29. Chansky K, Sculier JP, Crowley JJ, Giroux D, van Meerbeeck J, Goldstraw P. The International Association for the Study of Lung Cancer Staging Project. Prognostic factors and pathologic TNM stage in surgically managed non-small cell lung cancer. *J Thorac Oncol* 2009; 4: 792-801.

30. Rusch VW, Asamura H, Watanabe H, Giroux DJ, Rami-Porta R, Goldstraw P. The IASLC Lung Cancer Staging Project. A proposal for a new international lymph node map in the forthcoming seventh edition of the TNM classification for lung cancer. *J Thorac Oncol* 2009; 4: 568-577.

31. Travis WD, Brambilla E, Rami-Porta R, Vallieres E, Tsuboi M, Rusch V, et al. Visceral pleural invasion: pathologic criteria and use of elastic stains: proposals for the 7th edition of the TNM Classification for Lung Cancer. *J Thorac Oncol* 2008; 3: 1384-1390.

32. Goldstraw P. The 7th Edition of TNM for Lung Cancer: What now? *J Thorac Oncol* 2009; 4:671-673.

33. Giroux DJ, Rami-Porta R, Chansky K, Crowley JJ, Groome PA, Postmus PE, et al. The IASLC Lung Cancer Staging Project: data elements for the prospective project. *J Thorac Oncol* 2009;4:679-683.

34. Travis WD, Brambilla E, Muller-Hermelink HK, Harris CC. World Health Organisation Classification of Tumours: Pathology and Genetics of Tumors of the Lung, Pleura, Thymus and Heart. Lyon: IARC Press; 2004.

35. Lim E, Goldstraw P, Nicholson AG, Travis WD, Jett JR, Ferolla P, et al. Proceedings of the IASLC International Workshop on Advances in Neuroendocrine Tumors 2007. *J Thorac Oncol* 2008; 3: 1194-1201.

Acknowledgment: *Used with the permission of the Union for International Cancer Control (UICC), Geneva, Switzerland. The original source for this material is in Brierley JB, Gospodarowicz MK, Wittekind Ch, eds. UICC TNM Classification of Malignant Tumours, 8th edition (2017), published by John Wiley & Sons, Ltd, www.wiley.com.*

4

8th Edition of TNM for Lung Cancer

Introductory Notes

The classification applies to carcinomas of the lung including non-small cell and small cell carcinomas, and bronchopulmonary carcinoid tumours.

Each site is described under the following headings:

- Rules for classification with the procedures for assessing T, N, and M categories; additional methods may be used when they enhance the accuracy of appraisal before treatment
- Anatomical subsites where appropriate
- Definition of the regional lymph nodes
- TNM clinical classification
- pTNM pathological classification
- Stage
- Prognostic factors grid

Regional Lymph Nodes

The regional lymph nodes extend from the supraclavicular region to the diaphragm. Direct extension of the primary tumour into lymph nodes is classified as lymph node metastasis.

Lung
(ICD-O-3 C34)
Rules for Classification

The classification applies to carcinomas of the lung including non-small cell carcinomas, small cell carcinomas, and bronchopulmonary carcinoid tumours. It does not apply to sarcomas and other rare tumours.

Changes in this edition from the seventh edition are based upon recommendations from the International Association for the Study of Lung Cancer (IASLC) Staging Project (see references).[1-6]

There should be histological confirmation of the disease and division of cases by histological type.

The following are the procedures for assessing T, N, and M categories:

T categories Physical examination, imaging, endoscopy, and/or surgical exploration

N categories Physical examination, imaging, endoscopy, and/or surgical exploration

M categories Physical examination, imaging, and/or surgical exploration

Anatomical Subsites

1. Main bronchus (C34.0)
2. Upper lobe (C34.1)
3. Middle lobe (C34.2)
4. Lower lobe (C34.3)

Regional Lymph Nodes

The regional lymph nodes are the intrathoracic nodes (mediastinal, hilar, lobar, interlobar, segmental, and subsegmental), scalene, and supraclavicular lymph nodes.

TNM Clinical Classification

T – Primary Tumour

TX Primary tumour cannot be assessed, or tumour proven by the presence of malignant cells in sputum or bronchial washings but not visualized by imaging or bronchoscopy

T0 No evidence of primary tumour

Tis Carcinoma *in situ*[a]

T1 Tumour 3 cm or less in greatest dimension, surrounded by lung or visceral pleura, without bronchoscopic evidence of invasion more proximal than the lobar bronchus (i.e., not in the main bronchus)[b]

  T1mi Minimally invasive adenocarcinoma[c]

  T1a Tumour 1 cm or less in greatest dimension[b]

  T1b Tumour more than 1 cm but not more than 2 cm in greatest dimension[b]

  T1c Tumour more than 2 cm but not more than 3 cm in greatest dimension[b]

T2 Tumour more than 3 cm but not more than 5 cm; or tumour with *any* of the following features[d]

  • Involves main bronchus regardless of distance to the carina, but without involvement of the carina

      • Invades visceral pleura

      • Associated with atelectasis or obstructive pneumonitis that extends to the hilar region either involving part of or the entire lung

      T2a   Tumour more than 3 cm but not more than 4 cm in greatest dimension

      T2b   Tumour more than 4 cm but not more than 5 cm in greatest dimension

T3   Tumour more than 5 cm but not more than 7 cm in greatest dimension or one that directly invades any of the following: parietal pleura, chest wall (including superior sulcus tumours), phrenic nerve, parietal pericardium; or separate tumour nodule(s) in the same lobe as the primary

T4   Tumour more than 7 cm or of any size that invades any of the following: diaphragm, mediastinum, heart, great vessels, trachea, recurrent laryngeal nerve, oesophagus, vertebral body, carina; separate tumour nodule(s) in a different ipsilateral lobe to that of the primary

N – Regional Lymph Nodes

NX   Regional lymph nodes cannot be assessed

N0   No regional lymph node metastasis

N1   Metastasis in ipsilateral peribronchial and/or ipsilateral hilar lymph nodes and intrapulmonary nodes, including involvement by direct extension

N2   Metastasis in ipsilateral mediastinal and/or subcarinal lymph node(s)

N3   Metastasis in contralateral mediastinal, contralateral hilar, ipsilateral or contralateral scalene, or supraclavicular lymph node(s)

M – Distant Metastasis

M0   No distant metastasis

M1   Distant metastasis

      M1a   Separate tumour nodule(s) in a contralateral lobe; tumour with pleural or pericardial nodules or malignant pleural or pericardial effusion[e]

      M1b   Single extrathoracic metastasis in a single organ[f]

      M1c   Multiple extrathoracic metastasis in a single or multiple organs

Notes

[a] Tis includes adenocarcinoma *in situ* and squamous carcinoma *in situ*.

[b] The uncommon superficial spreading tumour of any size with its invasive component limited to the bronchial wall, which may extend proximal to the main bronchus, is also classified as T1a.

[c] Solitary adenocarcinoma (not more than 3 cm in greatest dimension), with a predominantly lepidic pattern and not more than 5 mm invasion in greatest dimension in any one focus.

[d] T2 tumours with these features are classified T2a if 4 cm or less, or if size cannot be determined and T2b if greater than 4 cm but not larger than 5 cm.

[e] Most pleural (pericardial) effusions with lung cancer are due to tumour. In a few patients,

however, multiple microscopic examinations of pleural (pericardial) fluid are negative for tumour, and the fluid is non-bloody and is not an exudate. Where these elements and clinical judgment dictate that the effusion is not related to the tumour, the effusion should be excluded as a staging descriptor.

[f]This includes involvement of a single non-regional node.

pTNM Pathological Classification

The pT and pN categories correspond to the T and N categories. For pM see page 59.

pN0 Histological examination of hilar and mediastinal lymphadenectomy specimen(s) will ordinarily include 6 or more lymph nodes/stations. Three of these nodes/stations should be mediastinal, including the subcarinal nodes and three from N1 nodes/stations. Labelling according to the IASLC chart and table of definitions given in the TNM Supplement is desirable. If all the lymph nodes examined are negative, but the number ordinarily examined is not met, classify as pN0.

Stage

Occult carcinoma	TX	N0	M0
Stage 0	Tis	N0	M0
Stage IA	T1	N0	M0
Stage IA1	T1mi	N0	M0
	T1a	N0	M0
Stage IA2	T1b	N0	M0
Stage IA3	T1c	N0	M0
Stage IB	T2a	N0	M0
Stage IIA	T2b	N0	M0
Stage IIB	T1a-c, T2a, b	N1	M0
	T3	N0	M0
Stage IIIA	T1a-c, T2a, b	N2	M0
	T3	N1	M0
	T4	N0, N1	M0
Stage IIIB	T1a-c, T2a, b	N3	M0
	T3, T4	N2	M0
Stage IIIC	T3, T4	N3	M0
Stage IV	Any T	Any N	M1
Stage IVA	Any T	Any N	M1a, M1b
Stage IVB	Any T	Any N	M1c

Prognostic Factors Grid – Non-Small Cell Lung Carcinoma

Prognostic factors in surgically resected NSCLC

Prognostic Factors	Tumour Related	Host Related	Environment Related
Essential	T category N category Extracapsular nodal extension	Weight loss Performance status	Resection margins Adequacy of mediastinal dissection
Additional	Histological type Grade Vessel invasion Tumour size	Gender Symptom burden	
New and promising	Molecular/ biological markers	Quality of life Marital status	

Source: *UICC Manual of Clinical Oncology*, Ninth Edition. Edited by Brian O'Sullivan, James D. Brierley, Anil K. D'Cruz, Martin F. Fey, Raphael Pollock, Jan B. Vermorken and Shao Hui Huang. © 2015 UICC. Published 2015 by John Wiley & Sons, Ltd.

Prognostic risk factors in advanced (locally-advanced or metastatic) NSCLC

Prognostic Factors	Tumour Related	Host Related	Environment Related
Essential	Stage Superior vena cava obstruction (SVCO) Oligometastatic disease Number of sites	Weight loss Performance status	Chemotherapy Targeted therapy
Additional	Number of metastatic sites Pleural effusion Liver metastasis Haemoglobin Lactate dehydrogenase (LDH) Albumin	Gender	
New and promising	Molecular/ biological markers	Quality of life Marital status Anxiety/ depression	

Source: *UICC Manual of Clinical Oncology*, Ninth Edition. Edited by Brian O'Sullivan, James D. Brierley, Anil K. D'Cruz, Martin F. Fey, Raphael Pollock, Jan B. Vermorken and Shao Hui Huang. © 2015 UICC. Published 2015 by John Wiley & Sons, Ltd.

Prognostic Factors Grid – Small Cell Lung Carcinoma

Prognostic risk factors in SCLC

Prognostic Factors	Tumour Related	Host Related	Environment Related
Essential	Stage	Performance status Age Comorbidity	Chemotherapy Thoracic radiotherapy Prophylactic cranial radiotherapy
Additional	LDH Alkaline phosphatase Cushing syndrome M0 – mediastinal involvement M1 – number of sites Brain or bone involvement White blood cell count (WBC)/platelet count		
New and promising	Molecular/ biological markers		

Source: *UICC Manual of Clinical Oncology*, Ninth Edition. Edited by Brian O'Sullivan, James D. Brierley, Anil K. D'Cruz, Martin F. Fey, Raphael Pollock, Jan B. Vermorken and Shao Hui Huang. © 2015 UICC. Published 2015 by John Wiley & Sons, Ltd.

References

1. Rami-Porta R, Bolejack V, Giroux DJ, et al. The IASLC Lung Cancer Staging Project: the new database to inform the 8th edition of the TNM classification of lung cancer. *J Thorac Oncol* 2014; 9: 1618–1624.
2. Rami-Porta R, Bolejack V, Crowley J, et al. The IASLC Lung Cancer Staging Project: proposals for the revisions of the T descriptors in the forthcoming 8th edition of the TNM classification for lung cancer. *J Thorac Oncol* 2015; 10: 990–1003.
3. Asamura H, Chansky K, Crowley J, et al. The IASLC Lung Cancer Staging Project: proposals for the revisions of the N descriptors in the forthcoming 8th edition of the TNM classification for lung cancer. *J Thorac Oncol* 2015; 10: 1675–1684.
4. Eberhardt WEE, Mitchell A, Crowley J, et al. The IASLC Lung Cancer Staging Project: proposals for the revisions of the M descriptors in the forthcoming 8th edition of the TNM classification for lung cancer. *J Thorac Oncol* 2015; 10: 1515–1522.
5. Goldstraw P, Chansky K, Crowley J, et al. The IASLC Lung Cancer Staging Project: proposals for the revision of the TNM stage grouping in the forthcoming (eighth) edition of the TNM classification for lung cancer. *J Thorac Oncol* 2016;11: 39–51.
6. Nicholson AG, Chansky K, Crowley J, et al. The IASLC Lung Cancer Staging Project: proposals for the revision of the clinical and pathological staging of small cell lung cancer in the forthcoming eighth edition of the TNM classification for lung cancer. *J Thorac Oncol* 2016;11: 300–311.

Executive Editor's Note: This chapter has been reprinted from Wittekind Ch, Compton CC, Brierley J, Sobin LH (eds) UICC TNM Supplement A Commentary on Uniform Use, fourth edition, John Wiley & Sons, Ltd., Oxford, 2012. Where needed, the text has been updated according to the 8th edition of the TNM classification of lung cancer.

5

Site-Specific Explanatory Notes for Lung Tumours

Rules for Classification

The classification applies to all types of carcinoma including non-small cell and small cell carcinoma and to broncho-pulmonary carcinoid tumours. It does not apply to sarcomas and other rare tumours.

Changes to the 7th edition are based upon recommendations from the IASLC Lung Cancer Staging Project.[1-12]

Clinical classification (Pre-treatment clinical classification), designated TNM (or cTNM), is essential to select and evaluate therapy. This is based on evidence acquired before treatment. Such evidence arises from physical examination, imaging (e.g., computed tomography and positron emission tomography), endoscopy (bronchoscopy or oesophagoscopy, with/without ultrasound directed biopsies (EBUS, EUS)), biopsy (including mediastinoscopy, mediastinotomy, thoracocentesis and video-assisted thoracoscopy), as well as surgical exploration, and other relevant examinations such as pleural/pericardial aspiration for cytology.

Pathological classification (post-surgical histopathological classification), designated pTNM, provides the most precise data to estimate prognosis and calculate end results. This is based on the evidence acquired before treatment, supplemented or modified by the additional evidence acquired from surgery and from pathological examination. The pathological assessment of the primary tumour (pT) entails a resection of the primary tumour, or biopsy adequate to evaluate the highest pT category. Removal of nodes adequate to validate the absence of regional lymph node metastasis is required for pN0. The pathological assessment of distant metastasis (pM) entails microscopic examination.

Pathologic staging depends on the proven anatomic extent of disease, whether or not the primary lesion has been completely removed. If a biopsied primary tumour technically cannot be removed, or when it is unreasonable to remove it, the criteria for pathologic classification and staging are satisfied without total removal of the primary cancer if: a) biopsy has confirmed a pT category and there is microscopical confirmation of nodal disease at any level (pN1-3), b) there is microscopical confirmation of the highest N category (pN3), or c) there is microscopical confirmation of pM1.

General Rule 3 states that clinical and pathological data may be combined when only partial information is available in either the pathological classification or the clinical classification, e.g. the classification of a case designated as cT1 pN2 cM1 or pT2 cN0 cM1 would be considered a clinical classification whilst in a case designated pT2 pN2 cM1, cT2 pN3 cM0 or cT2 cN0 pM1 case it would be appropriate to designate a pathological classification.

Histopathologic Type

Table 5.1. 2015 WHO Classification of Lung Tumours [a,b,c]

Histologic Type and Subtypes	ICDO Code
Epithelial tumours	
Adenocarcinoma	8140/3
Lepidic adenocarcinoma[e]	8250/3[d]
Acinar adenocarcinoma	8551/3[d]
Papillary adenocarcinoma	8260/3
Micropapillary adenocarcinoma[e]	8265/3
Solid adenocarcinoma	8230/3
Invasive mucinous adenocarcinoma[e]	8253/3[d]
Mixed invasive mucinous and nonmucinous adenocarcinoma	8254/3[d]
Colloid adenocarcinoma	8480/3
Fetal adenocarcinoma	8333/3
Enteric adenocarcinoma[e]	8144/3
Minimally invasive adenocarcinoma[e]	
Nonmucinous	8256/3[d]
Mucinous	8257/3[d]
Preinvasive lesions	
Atypical adenomatous hyperplasia	8250/0[d]
Adenocarcinoma in situ[e]	
Nonmucinous	8250/2[d]
Mucinous	8253/2[d]

continued on next page

Table 5.1. *(continued)*

Epithelial tumours (cont.)	
Squamous cell carcinoma	8070/3
Keratinizing squamous cell carcinoma[e]	8071/3
Nonkeratinizing squamous cell carcinoma[e]	8072/3
Basaloid squamous cell carcinoma[e]	8083/3
Preinvasive lesion	
Squamous cell carcinoma in situ	8070/2
Neuroendocrine tumours	
Small cell carcinoma	8041/3
Combined small cell carcinoma	8045/3
Large cell neuroendocrine carcinoma	8013/3
Combined large cell neuroendocrine carcinoma	8013/3
Carcinoid tumours	
Typical carcinoid tumour	8240/3
Atypical carcinoid tumour	8249/3
Preinvasive lesion	
Diffuse idiopathic pulmonary neuroendocrine cell hyperplasia	8040/0[d]
Large cell carcinoma	8012/3
Adenosquamous carcinoma	8560/3
Sarcomatoid carcinomas	
Pleomorphic carcinoma	8022/3
Spindle cell carcinoma	8032/3
Giant cell carcinoma	8031/3
Carcinosarcoma	8980/3
Pulmonary blastoma	8972/3
Other and unclassified carcinomas	
Lymphoepithelioma-like carcinoma	8082/3
NUT carcinoma[e]	8023/3[d]
Salivary gland-type tumours	
Mucoepidermoid carcinoma	8430/3
Adenoid cystic carcinoma	8200/3
Epithelial-myoepithelial carcinoma	8562/3
Pleomorphic adenoma	8940/0
Papillomas	
Squamous cell papilloma	8052/0
Exophytic	8052/0
Inverted	8053/0

continued on next page

Table 5.1. *(continued)*

Histologic Type and Subtypes	ICDO Code
Neuroendocrine tumours (cont.)	
Glandular papilloma	8260/0
Mixed squamous and glandular papilloma	8560/0
Adenomas	
Sclerosing pneumocytoma[e]	8832/0
Alveolar adenoma	8251/0
Papillary adenoma	8260/0
Mucinous cystadenoma	8470/0
Mucous gland adenoma	8480/0
Mesenchymal tumours	
Pulmonary hamartoma	8992/0[d]
Chondroma	9220/0
PEComatous tumours[e]	
Lymphangioleiomyomatosis	9174/1
PEComa, benign[e]	8714/0
Clear cell tumour	8005/0
PEComa, malignant[e]	8714/3
Congenital peribronchial myofibroblastic tumour	8827/1
Diffuse pulmonary lymphangiomatosis	
Inflammatory myofibroblastic tumour	8825/1
Epithelioid hemangioendothelioma	9133/3
Pleuropulmonary blastoma	8973/3
Synovial sarcoma	9040/3
Pulmonary artery intimal sarcoma	9137/3
Pulmonary myxoid sarcoma with EWSR1–CREB1 translocation[e]	8842/3[d]
Myoepithelial tumours[e]	
Myoepithelioma	8982/0
Myoepithelial carcinoma	8982/3
Lymphohistiocytic tumours	
Extranodal marginal zone lymphomas of mucosa-associated lymphoid tissue (MALT lymphoma)	9699/3
Diffuse large cell lymphoma	9680/3
Lymphomatoid granulomatosis	9766/1
Intravascular large B cell lymphoma[e]	9712/3
Pulmonary Langerhans cell histiocytosis	9751/1
Erdheim–Chester disease	9750/1

continued on next page

Table 5.1. *(continued)*

Tumours of ectopic origin	
Germ cell tumours	
Teratoma, mature	9080/0
Teratoma, immature	9080/1
Intrapulmonary thymoma	8580/3
Melanoma	8270/3
Meningioma, NOS	9530/0
Metastatic tumours	

[a]*The morphology codes are from the ICDO (Fritz A, Percy C, Jack A, et al. International Classification of Diseases for Oncology. 3rd ed. Geneva: World Health Organization (WHO), 2000). Behavior is coded /0 for benign tumors, /1 for unspecified, borderline or uncertain behavior, /2 for carcinoma in situ and grade III intraepithelial neoplasia, and /3 for malignant tumors.*

[b]*The classification is modified from the previous WHO classification[3] taking into account changes in our understanding of these lesions.*

[c]*This table is reproduced from the 2015 WHO Classification by Travis WD, Brambilla E, Burke AP, Marx A, Nicholson AG. WHO Classification of Tumours of the Lung, Pleura, Thymus and Heart. Lyon: International Agency for Research on Cancer, 2015.*

[d]*These new codes were approved by the International Agency on Cancer Research/WHO Committee for ICDO.*

[e]*New terms changed or entities added since 2004 WHO Classification by Travis WD, Brambilla E, Müller-Hermelink HK, Harris CC. Pathology and Genetics: Tumours of the Lung, Pleura, Thymus and Heart. Lyon: IARC, 2004.'*

LCNEC, large cell neuroendocrine carcinoma, WHO, World Health Organization; ICDO International Classification of Diseases for Oncology.

From: Travis WD, Brambilla E, Nicholson AG et al. The 2015 World Health Organization Classification of Lung Tumors. Impact of genetic, clinical and radiologic advances since the 2004 classification. J Thorac Oncol 2015; 10: 1243-1260. Used with permission.[13]

Summary Lung

TX   Primary tumour cannot be assessed, or tumour proven by the presence of malignant cells in sputum or bronchial washings but not visualized by imaging or bronchoscopy

T0   No evidence of primary tumour

Tis   Carcinoma *in situ*: Tis (AIS) for adenocarcinoma *in situ*; Tis (SCIS) for squamous cell carcinoma *in situ*.

T1   Tumour 3 cm or less in greatest dimension, surrounded by lung or visceral pleura, without bronchoscopic evidence of invasion more proximal than the lobar bronchus (i.e., not in the main bronchus). The uncommon superficial spreading tumour of any size with its invasive component limited to the bronchial wall, which may extend proximal to the main bronchus, is also classified as T1a.

   T1mi Minimally invasive adenocarcinoma

   T1a Tumour 1 cm or less in greatest dimension

   T1b Tumour more than 1 cm but not more than 2 cm in greatest dimension

   T1c Tumour more than 2 cm but not more than 3 cm in greatest dimension

T2 Tumour more than 3 cm but not more than 5 cm; or tumour with any of the following features. T2 tumours with these features are classified T2a if 4 cm or less, or if size cannot be determined; and T2b if greater than 4 cm but not larger than 5 cm.

- Involves main bronchus regardless of distance to the carina, but without involving the carina
- Invades visceral pleura
- Associated with atelectasis or obstructive pneumonitis that extends to the hilar region, either involving part of the lung or the entire lung

T2a Tumour more than 3 cm but not more than 4 cm in greatest dimension

T2b Tumour more than 4 cm but not more than 5 cm in greatest dimension

T3 Tumour more than 5 cm but not more than 7 cm in greatest dimension or one that directly invades any of the following: parietal pleura (PL3), chest wall (including superior sulcus tumours), phrenic nerve, parietal pericardium; or associated separate tumour nodule(s) in the same lobe as the primary

T4 Tumour more than 7 cm or one that invades any of the following: diaphragm, mediastinum, heart, great vessels, trachea, recurrent laryngeal nerve, oesophagus, vertebral body, carina; separate tumour nodule(s) in a different ipsilateral lobe to that of the primary

N – Regional Lymph Nodes

NX Regional lymph nodes cannot be assessed

N0 No regional lymph node metastasis

N1 Metastasis in ipsilateral peribronchial and/or ipsilateral hilar lymph nodes and intrapulmonary nodes, including involvement by direct extension

N2 Metastasis in ipsilateral mediastinal and/or subcarinal lymph node(s)

N3 Metastasis in contralateral mediastinal, contralateral hilar, ipsilateral or contralateral scalene, or supraclavicular lymph node(s)

M – Distant Metastasis

M0 No distant metastasis

M1 Distant metastasis

M1a Separate tumour nodule(s) in a contralateral lobe; tumour with pleural nodules or malignant pleural or pericardial effusion. Most pleural (pericardial) effusions with lung cancer are due to tumour. In a few patients, however, multiple microscopic examinations of pleural (pericardial) fluid are negative for tumour, and the fluid is non-bloody and is not an exudate. Where these elements and clinical judgment dictate that the effusion is not related to the tumour, the effusion should be excluded as a staging descriptor.

M1b Single extrathoracic metastasis in a single organ and involvement of a single distant (non-regional) node

M1c Multiple extrathoracic metastases in one or several organs

T Classification

1. Invasion of visceral pleura (T2) is defined as "invasion beyond the elastic layer including invasion to the visceral pleural surface". The use of elastic stains is recommended when this feature is not clear on routine histology.[14] See Chapter 7 for additional information under "New TNM classifications for testing" and Figure 1 of that chapter.

2. Tumour with direct invasion of an adjacent lobe, across the fissure or by direct extension at a point where the fissure is deficient, should be classified as T2a unless other criteria assign a higher T category.

3. Invasion of phrenic nerve is classified as T3.

4. Vocal cord paralysis (resulting from involvement of the recurrent branch of the vagus nerve), superior vena caval obstruction, or compression of the trachea or oesophagus may be related to direct extension of the primary tumour or to lymph node involvement. If associated with direct extension of the primary tumour a classification of T4 is recommended. If the primary tumour is peripheral, vocal cord paralysis is usually related to the presence of N2 disease and should be classified as such.

5. T4: the "great vessels" are
   - Aorta
   - Superior vena cava
   - Inferior vena cava
   - Main pulmonary artery (pulmonary trunk)
   - Intrapericardial portions of the right and left pulmonary artery
   - Intrapericardial portions of the superior and inferior right and left pulmonary veins

   Invasion of more distal branches does not qualify for classification as T4

6. The designation of "Pancoast" tumour relates to the symptom complex or syndrome caused by a tumour arising in the superior sulcus of the lung that involves the inferior branches of the brachial plexus (C8 and/or T1) and, in some cases, the stellate ganglion. Some superior sulcus tumours are more anteriorly located, and cause fewer neurological symptoms but encase the subclavian vessels. The extent of disease varies in these tumours, and they should be classified according to the established rules. If there is evidence of invasion of the vertebral body or spinal canal, encasement of the subclavian vessels,

or unequivocal involvement of the superior branches of the brachial plexus (C8 or above), the tumour is then classified as T4. If no criteria for T4 disease are present, the tumour is classified as T3.

7. Direct extension to parietal pericardium is classified T3 and to visceral pericardium, T4.

8. Tumour extending to rib is classified as T3.

9. The uncommon superficial spreading tumour of any size with its invasive component limited to the bronchial wall, which may extend proximal to the main bronchus, is classified as T1a.

10. The classification of additional tumour nodules in lung cancer depends upon their histological appearances. a) In most situations in which additional tumour nodules are found in association with a lung primary these are metastatic nodules, with identical histological appearances to that of the primary tumour. If limited to the lobe of the primary tumour such tumours are classified as T3, when found in other ipsilateral lobes are designated as T4 and if found in the contralateral lung are designated M1a. b) Multiple tumours may be considered to be synchronous primaries if they are of different histological cell types. Multiple tumours of similar histological appearance should only be considered to be synchronous primary tumours if in the opinion of the pathologist, based on features such as differences in morphology, immunohistochemistry and/or molecular studies, or, in the case of squamous cancers, are associated with carcinoma in situ, they represent differing sub-types of the same histopathological cell type. Such cases should also have no evidence of mediastinal nodal metastases or of nodal metastases within a common nodal drainage. These circumstances are most commonly encountered when dealing with either bronchioloalveolar carcinomas or adenocarcinomas of mixed subtype with a bronchioloalveolar component. Multiple synchronous primary tumours should be staged separately. The highest T category and stage of disease should be assigned and the multiplicity or the number of tumours should be indicated in parenthesis, e.g. T2(m) or T2. This distinction may require histopathological confirmation of cell type from more than one tumour nodule, where clinically appropriate.

Executive Editor's Note: *Please, see Chapter 8 for additional recommendations on how to classify lung cancers with multiple lesions.*

In the above classification lung differs from other sites in the application of General Rule 5 as the classification of additional tumour nodules applies not only to grossly recognizable tumours but also those that are microscopic or otherwise only discovered on pathological examination, a not unusual finding in lung cancer.

11. Invasion into mediastinal fat is T4. However, if such invasion is clearly limited to fat within the hilum, classification as T2a or T2b is appropriate, depending upon size, unless other features dictate a higher T category.

N Classification

1. The regional lymph nodes are the intrathoracic, scalene, and supraclavicular nodes.
2. The International Association for the Study of Lung Cancer (IASLC) lymph node definitions are now the recommended means of describing regional lymph node involvement for lung cancers[15] (see Table 5.2 and Figure 5.1 and 5.2).In this nomenclature ipsilateral or contralateral node involvement in #1 would be classified as N3. Involvement of mediastinal nodes, if limited to the midline stations or ipsilateral stations (#2-9), would be classified as N2. Involvement of #10-14 if ipsilateral would be classified as N1. Contralateral involvement of # 2, 4, 5, 6, 8, 9, 10-14 would be classified as N3.
3. Direct extension of the primary tumour into lymph nodes is classified as lymph node metastasis.
4. The IASLC nodal chart has been adopted as the new international chart for the documentation of nodal stations at clinical or pathological staging where detailed assessment of nodes has been made, usually by invasive techniques or at thoracotomy. The concept of nodal zones was suggested in the 7th edition of the TNM classification of lung cancer as a simpler, more utilitarian system for clinical staging where surgical exploration of lymph nodes has not been performed. An exploratory analysis suggested that nodal extent could be grouped into three categories with differing prognoses: i) involvement of a single N1 zone, designated as N1a, ii) involvement of more than one N1 zone, designated as N1b, or a single N2 zone, designated N2a, and iii) involvement of more than one N2 zone, designated as N2b. It was suggested that radiologists, clinicians and oncologists use the classification prospectively, where more detailed data on nodal stations is not available, to assess the utility of such a classification for future revision.

Executive Editor's Note: For the 8th edition, quantification of nodal disease has been based on the number of nodal stations involved. The survival analyses performed on patients whose tumours were resected and had an adequate intraoperative nodal evaluation revealed four categories with different prognosis: i) involvement of a single N1 station, designated as N1a, ii) involvement of more than one N1 station, designated as N1b, or involvement of one N2 station without N1 disease (skip metastasis), designated as N2a1, iii) involvement of one N2 station with N1 disease, designated as N2a2, and iv) involvement of more than one N2 station, designated N2b. From the

Table 5.2. IASLC Nodal Definitions.

Nodal station	Description	Definition
#1 (Left/Right)	Low cervical, supraclavicular and sternal notch nodes	Upper border: lower margin of cricoid cartilage Lower border: clavicles bilaterally and, in the midline, the upper border of the manubrium **#L1 and #R1 limited by the midline of the trachea.**

#2 (Left/Right)	Upper paratracheal nodes	2R: Upper border: apex of lung and pleural space and, in the midline, the upper border of the manubrium
		   Lower border: intersection of caudal margin of innominate vein with the trachea
		2L: Upper border: apex of the lung and pleural space and, in the midline, the upper border of the manubrium
		   Lower border: superior border of the aortic arch
		As for #4, in #2 the oncologic midline is along the left lateral border of the trachea.

#3	Pre-vascular and retrotracheal nodes	3a: Prevascular **On the right** upper border: apex of chest lower border: level of carina anterior border: posterior aspect of sternum posterior border: anterior border of superior vena cava **On the left** upper border: apex of chest lower border: level of carina anterior border: posterior aspect of sternum posterior border: left carotid artery 3p: Retrotracheal upper border: apex of chest lower border: carina
#4 (Left/Right)	Lower paratracheal nodes	4R: includes right paratracheal nodes, and pretracheal nodes extending to the left lateral border of trachea upper border: intersection of caudal margin of innominate vein with the trachea lower border: lower border of azygos vein 4L: includes nodes to the left of the left lateral border of the trachea, medial to the ligamentum arteriosum upper border: upper margin of the aortic arch lower border: upper rim of the left main pulmonary artery

continued on next page

#5	Subaortic (aorto-pulmonary window)	Subaortic lymph nodes lateral to the ligamentum arteriosum upper border: the lower border of the aortic arch lower border: upper rim of the left main pulmonary artery
#6	Para-aortic nodes (ascending aorta or phrenic)	Lymph nodes anterior and lateral to the ascending aorta and aortic arch upper border: a line tangential to the upper border of the aortic arch lower border: the lower border of the aortic arch
#7	Subcarinal nodes	upper border: the carina of the trachea lower border: the upper border of the lower lobe bronchus on the left; the lower border of the bronchus intermedius on the right
#8 (Left/Right)	Para-oesophageal nodes (below carina)	Nodes lying adjacent to the wall of the oesophagus and to the right or left of the midline, excluding subcarinal nodes upper border: the upper border of the lower lobe bronchus on the left; the lower border of the bronchus intermedius on the right lower border: the diaphragm
#9 (Left/Right)	Pulmonary ligament nodes	Nodes lying within the pulmonary ligament upper border: the inferior pulmonary vein lower border: the diaphragm
#10 (Left/Right)	Hilar nodes	Includes nodes immediately adjacent to the mainstem bronchus and hilar vessels including the proximal portions of the pulmonary veins and main pulmonary artery upper border: the lower rim of the azygos vein on the right; upper rim of the pulmonary artery on the left lower border: interlobar region bilaterally
#11	Interlobar nodes	Between the origin of the lobar bronchi *#11s: between the upper lobe bronchus and bronchus intermedius on the right *#11i: between the middle and lower lobe bronchi on the right * optional sub-categories
#12	Lobar nodes	Adjacent to the lobar bronchi
#13	Segmental nodes	Adjacent to the segmental bronchi
#14	Sub-segmental nodes	Adjacent to the subsegmental bronchi

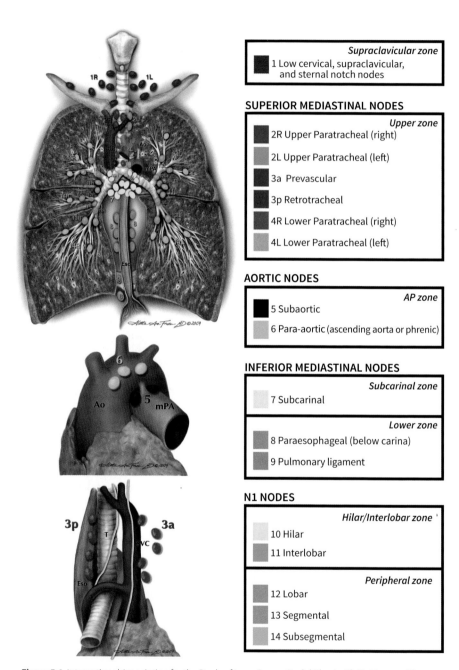

Supraclavicular zone

■ 1 Low cervical, supraclavicular, and sternal notch nodes

SUPERIOR MEDIASTINAL NODES

Upper zone

■ 2R Upper Paratracheal (right)

■ 2L Upper Paratracheal (left)

■ 3a Prevascular

■ 3p Retrotracheal

■ 4R Lower Paratracheal (right)

■ 4L Lower Paratracheal (left)

AORTIC NODES

AP zone

■ 5 Subaortic

■ 6 Para-aortic (ascending aorta or phrenic)

INFERIOR MEDIASTINAL NODES

Subcarinal zone

■ 7 Subcarinal

Lower zone

■ 8 Paraesophageal (below carina)

■ 9 Pulmonary ligament

N1 NODES

Hilar/Interlobar zone

■ 10 Hilar

■ 11 Interlobar

Peripheral zone

■ 12 Lobar

■ 13 Segmental

■ 14 Subsegmental

Figure 5.1 International Association for the Study of Lung Cancer Nodal Chart with Stations and Zones. Copyright ©2008 Aletta Ann Frazier, MD.

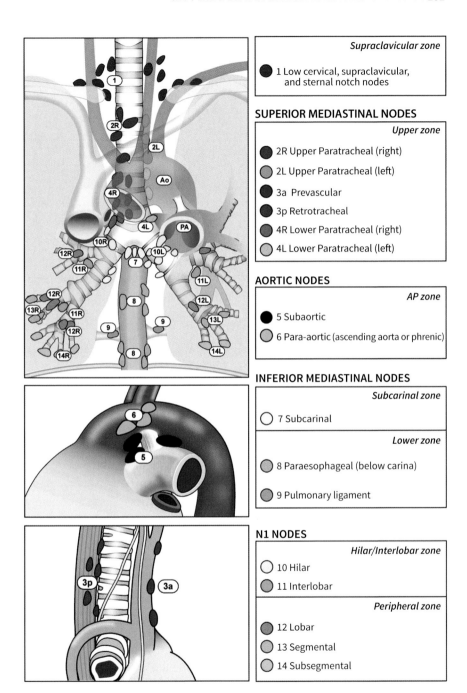

Figure 5.2 International Association for the Study of Lung Cancer Nodal Chart with Stations and Zones. Copyright ©2009 Memorial Sloan-Kettering Cancer Center.

analyses of nodal zones and stations, it is evident that the amount of nodal disease has prognostic impact. It is suggested that quantification of nodal disease be made with the available methods at clinical staging, and with systematic nodal dissection at the time of lung resection, either open or video-assisted. Quantifying nodal disease assists physicians in refining prognosis, and in planning therapy and follow-up.

M Classification

1. Pleural/pericardial effusions are classified as M1a, Most pleural (pericardial) effusions with lung cancer are due to tumour. In a few patients, however, multiple microscopical examinations of pleural (pericardial) fluid are negative for tumour, and the fluid is non-bloody and is not an exudate. Where these elements and clinical judgment dictate that the effusion is not related to the tumour, the effusion should be excluded as a descriptor.
2. Tumour foci in the ipsilateral parietal and visceral pleura that are discontinuous from direct pleural invasion by the primary tumour are classified M1a.
3. Pericardial effusion/pericardial nodules are classified as M1a, the same as pleural effusion/nodules.
4. Separate tumour nodules of similar histological appearance are classed as M1a if in the contralateral lung (vide supra regarding synchronous primaries).
5. Distant metastases are classified as M1b if single and M1c if multiple in one or in several organs.
6. Discontinuous tumours outside the parietal pleura in the chest wall or in the diaphragm are classified M1b or M1c depending on the number of lesions.
7. In cases classified as M1b and M1c due to distant metastases it is important to document all of the sites of metastatic disease, whether the sites are solitary or multiple and in addition if the metastases at each site are solitary or multiple.

V Classification

In the lung, arterioles are frequently invaded by cancers. For this reason the V classification is applicable to indicate vascular invasion, whether venous or arteriolar.

Small Cell Carcinoma

The TNM classification and stage grouping should be applied to small cell lung cancer (SCLC). TNM is of significance for prognosis of small cell carcinoma,[6] and has the advantage of providing a uniform detailed classification of tumour spread. TNM should be used when undertaking trials in SCLC. The former categories "limited" and "extensive" for small cell carcinoma have been inconsistently defined and used.

Broncho-Pulmonary Carcinoid Tumours

The TNM classification and stage groupings should be applied to carcinoid tumours, typical and atypical variants.[16]

Isolated Tumour Cells (ITC)

Isolated tumour cells (ITC) are single tumour cells or small clusters of cells not more than 0.2 mm in greatest dimension that are detected by routine histological stains, immunohistochemistry or molecular methods. Cases with ITC in lymph nodes or at distant sites should be classified as N0 or M0, respectively. The same applies to cases with findings suggestive of tumour cells or their components by nonmorphologic techniques such as flow cytometry or DNA analysis.

The following classification of ITC may be used:

N0	No regional lymph node metastasis histologically, no special examination for ITC
N0(i-)	No regional lymph node metastasis histologically, negative morphological findings for ITC
N0(i+)	No regional lymph node metastasis histologically, positive morphological findings for ITC
N0(mol-)	No regional lymph node metastasis histologically, negative nonmorphological findings for ITC
N0(mol+)	No regional lymph node metastasis histologically, positive nonmorphological findings for ITC

Expansion of the R Classification
RX   Presence of residual tumour cannot be assessed
R0   Complete resection
All of the following are satisfied:
a)   Resection margins confirmed to be clear on microscopy
b)   Six nodes/nodal stations removed/sampled for histological examination. These should include three nodes/stations from the mediastinum, one of which should be subcarinal node #7 and three nodes/stations from the hilum or other N1 locations*

R1(cy+)
The requirements for R0 have been met, but pleural lavage cytology (PLC) is positive for malignant cells.

A recent meta-analysis[17] has confirmed that PLC, undertaken immediately on thoracotomy and shown to be positive for cancer cells, has an adverse and independent prognostic impact following complete resection. Such patients may be candidates for adjuvant chemotherapy. Surgeons and pathologists are encouraged to undertake this simple addition to intra-operative staging and collect data on PLC+ve and PLC-ve cases. Where the resection fulfills all of the requirements for classification as a complete resection, R0, but PLC has been performed and is positive, the resection should be classified as R1(cy+).

R1(is)
The requirements for R0 have been met, but *in situ* carcinoma is found at the bronchial resection margin.

R1 Microscopic incomplete resection
Microscopic evidence of residual disease at any of the following sites:
a) Resection margins
b) Extracapsular extension at margins of resected nodes
c) Positive cytology of pleural/pericardial effusions (R1(cy+))

R2 Macroscopic incomplete resection
Macroscopic evidence of residual disease at any of the following sites:
a) Resection margins
b) Extracapsular extension at margins of resected nodes
c) Positive nodes not resected at surgery
d) Pleural/pericardial nodules

*If all resected/sampled lymph nodes are negative, but the number ordinarily included in a lymphadenectomy specimen is not met, classify as pN0. If resection has been performed, and otherwise fulfils the requirements for complete resection, it should be classified as R0.

A new category, '**R0(un)**', is proposed to document those other features that fall within the proposed category of '**uncertain resection**', i.e. no macroscopic or microscopic evidence of residual disease but any of the following reservations applies:
i)   Nodal assessment has been based on less than the number of nodes/stations recommended for complete resection
ii) The highest mediastinal node removed/sampled is positive

References
1. Rami-Porta R, Bolejack V, Giroux DJ et al. The IASLC lung cancer staging project: the new database to inform the eighth edition of the TNM classification of lung cancer. *J Thorac Oncol* 2014; 9: 1618-1624.
2. Rami-Porta R, Bolejack V, Crowley J et al. The IASLC lung cancer staging project: proposals for the revisions of the T descriptors in the forthcoming 8th edition of the TNM classification for lung cancer. *J Thorac Oncol* 2015; 10: 990-1003.

3. Asamura H, Chansky K, Crowley J et al. The IASLC lung cancer staging project: proposals for the revisions of the N descriptors in the forthcoming 8th edition of the TNM classification for lung cancer. *J Thorac Oncol* 2015; 10: 1675-1684.

4. Eberhardt WEE, Mitchell A, Crowley J et al. The IASLC lung cancer staging project: proposals for the revisions of the M descriptors in the forthcoming 8th edition of the TNM classification for lung cancer. *J Thorac Oncol* 2015; 10: 1515-1522.

5. Goldstraw P, Chansky K, Crowley J et al. The IASLC lung cancer staging project: proposals for the revision of the stage grouping in the forthcoming (8th) edition of the TNM classification of lung cancer. *J Thorac Oncol* 2016; 11: 39-51.

6. Nicholson AG, Chansky K, Crowley J et al. The IASLC lung cancer staging project: proposals for the revision of the clinical and pathologic staging of small cell lung cancer in the forthcoming eighth edition of the TNM classification for lung cancer. *J Thorac Oncol* 2016; 11: 300-311.

7. Travis WD, Asamura H, Bankier A et al. The IASLC Lung Cancer Staging Project: proposals for coding T categories for subsolid nodules and assessment of tumor size in part-solid tumors in the forthcoming eighth edition of the TNM classification of lung cancer. *J Thorac Oncol* 2016; 11: 1204-1223.

8. Detterbeck FC, Franklin WA, Nicholson AG et al. The IASLC Lung Cancer Staging Project: proposed criteria to distinguish separate primary lung cancers from metastatic foci in patients with two lung tumors in the forthcoming eighth edition of the TNM classification for lung cancer. *J Thorac Oncol* 2016; 11: 651-665.

9. Detterbeck FC, Bolejack V, Arenberg DA et al. The IASLC Lung Cancer Staging Project: proposals for the classification of lung cancer with separate tumor nodules in the forthcoming eighth edition of the TNM classification for lung cancer. *J Thorac Oncol* 2016; 11: 681-692.

10. Detterbeck FC, Marom EM, Arenberg DA et al. The IASLC Lung Cancer Staging Project: proposals for the application of TNM staging rules to lung cancer presenting as multiple nodules with ground glass or lepidic features or a pneumonic-type of involvement in the forthcoming eighth edition of the TNM classification. *J Thorac Oncol* 2016; 11: 666-680.

11. Detterbeck FC, Nicholson AG, Franklin WA et al. The IASLC Lung Cancer Staging Project: proposals for revisions of the classification of lung cancers with multiple pulmonary sites of involvement in the forthcoming eighth edition of the TNM classification. *J Thorac Oncol* 2016; 11: 639-650.

12. Detterbeck F, Groome P, Bolejack V et al. The IASLC Lung Cancer Staging Project: methodology and validation used in the development of proposals for revision if the stage classification of non-small cell lung cancer in the forthcoming (eighth) edition of the TNM classification of lung cancer. *J Thorac Oncol* 2016; 11: 1433-1446.

13. Travis WD, Brambilla E, Nicholson AG et al. The 2015 World Health Organization Classification of Lung Tumors. Impact of genetic, clinical and radiologic advances since the 2004 classification. *J Thorac Oncol* 2015; 10: 1243-1260.

14. Travis WD, Brambilla E, Rami-Porta R, et al. Visceral pleural invasion: Pathologic criteria and use of elastic stains: Proposals for the 7th edition of the TNM classification for lung cancer. *J Thorac Oncol* 2008; 3: 1384-1390.

15. Rusch VW, Asamura H, Watanabe H, Giroux DJ, Rami-Porta R, Goldstraw P. The IASLC Lung Cancer Staging Project. A proposal for a new international lymph node map in the forthcoming seventh edition of the TNM classification for lung cancer. *J Thorac Oncol* 2009; 4: 568-577.

16. Travis WD, Giroux DJ, Chansky K, et al. The IASLC Lung Cancer Project: proposals for the inclusion of broncho-pulmonary carcinoid tumors in the forthcoming (seventh) edition of the TNM classification for lung cancer. *J Thorac Oncol* 2008; 3: 1213-1223.

17. Lim E, Clough R, Goldstraw P et al. Impact of positive pleural lavage cytology on survival of patients having lung resection for non-small-cell lung cancer: An international individual patient data meta-analysis. *J Thorac Cardiovasc Surg* 2010; 139: 1441-1446.

Executive Editor's Note: This chapter has been reprinted from Wittekind Ch, Compton CC, Brierley J, Sobin LH (eds) UICC TNM Supplement A Commentary on Uniform Use, fourth edition, John Wiley & Sons, Ltd., Oxford, 2012. Where needed, the text has been updated according to the 8th edition of the TNM classification of lung cancer.

6

Site-Specific Recommendations for pT and pN Categories

pT – Primary Tumour

The pathological assessment of the primary tumour (pT) entails resection of the primary tumours sufficient to evaluate the highest pT category

pT3 or less

Pathological examination of the primary carcinoma shows *no gross tumour* at the margins of resection (with or without microscopic involvement). pT3 may include additional tumour nodule(s) of similar histological appearance in the lobe of the primary tumour.

pT4

Microscopic confirmation of invasion of any of the following: diaphragm, mediastinum, heart, great vessels, trachea, recurrent laryngeal nerve, oesophagus, vertebral body, carina *or* microscopic confirmation of separate tumour nodule(s) of similar histological appearance in another ipsilateral lobe (not the lobe of the primary tumour)

pN – Regional Lymph Nodes

There are no evidence-based guidelines regarding the number of lymph nodes to be removed at surgery for adequate staging. However, adequate N staging is generally considered to include sampling or dissection of lymph nodes from stations 2R, 4R, 7, 10R and 11R for right-sided tumours, and stations 5, 6, 7, 10L and 11L for left-sided tumours. Station 9 lymph nodes should also be evaluated for lower lobe tumours. The more peripheral lymph nodes at stations 12-14 are usually evaluated by the pathologist in lobectomy or pneumonectomy specimens but may be separately removed when sublobar resections (e.g. segmentectomy) are performed. These should be labelled in accordance with the IASLC chart and table of definitions[1] (see table and map on pages 98-101).

The UICC recommends that at least six lymph nodes/stations be removed/ sampled and confirmed on histology to be free of disease to confer pN0 status. Three of these nodes/stations should be mediastinal, including the subcarinal nodes (#7) and three from N1 nodes/stations.

If all resected/sampled lymph nodes are negative, but the number recommended is not met, classify as pN0. If resection has been performed, and otherwise fulfils the requirements for complete resection, it should be classified as R0.

pN1
Microscopic confirmation of metastasis in ipsilateral peribronchial and/or ipsilateral hilar lymph nodes and intrapulmonary nodes, including involvement by direct extension.

pN2
Microscopic confirmation of metastasis in ipsilateral mediastinal and/or subcarinal lymph node(s).

pN3
Microscopic confirmation of metastasis in contralateral mediastinal, contralateral hilar, ipsilateral or contraletaral scalene or supraclavicular lymph node(s).

Reference
1. Rusch VW, Asamura H, Watanabe H, Giroux DJ, Rami-Porta R, Goldstraw P. The IASLC lung cancer staging project. A proposal for a new international lymph node map in the forthcoming seventh edition of the TNM classification for lung cancer. *J Thorac Oncol* 2009; 4: 568-577

7

New TNM Classifications for Testing

a) Concerns have been expressed that the definition of complete resection conferring R0 status is too imprecise and that the application of General Rule 4 does not allow one to assess several features which may represent minimal residual disease and have an adverse prognostic influence. The category **"Uncertain Resection"** has been proposed[1] for testing. There is extant a category **"R1(is)"** which is applicable when the requirements for R0 have been met, but *in situ* carcinoma is found at the bronchial resection margin. Similarly category **"R1(cy+)"** is appropriate when the requirements for R0 have been met, but Pleural Lavage Cytology (PLC) is positive for malignant cells (v.i.). The wider use of these descriptors is encouraged to facilitate data collection and to assess the prognostic impact of these features following resection. A new category, **"R0(un)"**, is proposed to document those other features that fall within the proposed category of **"Uncertain Resection"**, i.e. no macroscopic or microscopic evidence of residual disease but any of the following reservations applies:

   i) Nodal assessment has been based on less than the number of nodes/stations recommended for complete resection.
   ii) The highest mediastinal node removed/sampled is positive.

b) A recent meta-analysis[2] has confirmed that pleural lavage cytology (PLC), undertaken immediately on thoracotomy and shown to be positive for cancer cells, has an adverse and independent prognostic impact following complete resection. Such patients may be candidates for adjuvant chemotherapy. Surgeons and pathologists are encouraged to undertake this simple addition to intra-operative staging and collect data on PLC+ve and PLC-ve cases. Where the resection fulfills all of the requirements for classification as a Complete Resection, R0, but PLC has been performed and is positive the resection should be classified as R1(cy+).

c) A standardized definition of visceral pleural invasion (VPI) has been incorporated into the 7th edition of TNM and maintained in the 8th edition. Recommendations included on the use of elastic stains in the determination of VPI.[3] It is important that data be collected using this definition so that the utility of this pT2 descriptor can be assessed more accurately in future revisions. A sub-classification has been proposed[3] based upon a system published by the Japan Lung Cancer Society[4] and by Hammar[5] (Figure 7.1). It is proposed that the PL category be used to describe the pathological extent of pleural invasion:

PL0 tumour within the subpleural lung parenchyma or invades superficially into the pleural connective tissue beneath the elastic layer.*

PL1 tumour invades beyond the elastic layer.

PL2 tumour invades to the pleural surface.

PL3 tumour invades into any component of the parietal pleura.

*Note: In the TNM 7th and 8th editions, PL0 is not regarded as a T descriptor and the T category should be assigned on other features. PL1 or PL2 indicate "visceral pleural invasion" i.e. T2a. PL3 indicates invasion of the parietal pleura, i.e. T3.

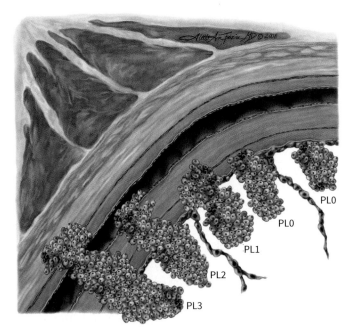

Figure 7.1. Visceral pleural invasion. Copyright ©2016 Aletta Ann Frazier, MD.

It is recommended that pathologists prospectively collect data based upon these sub-categories to facilitate future revisions of TNM.

d) There are suggestions that the depth of chest wall invasion may influence prognosis following resection of lung cancer. A sub-classification has been proposed, based upon the histopathological findings of the resection specimen, dividing such pT3 tumours into pT3a if invasion is limited to the parietal pleura (PL 3), pT3b if invasion involves the endothoracic fascia, and pT3c if invasion involves the rib or soft tissue. Pathologists are encouraged to collect this information prospectively to facilitate analysis and future revisions.

e) Imaging evidence of lymphangitis carcinomatosis is usually a contraindication to surgical treatment. The "L" category which is used to assess "lymphatic invasion" is therefore not applicable. The radiological extent of lymphangitis is thought to be of prognostic importance. An exploratory analysis of this feature is proposed using a "cLy" category in which cLy0 indicates that radiological evidence of lymphangitis is absent, cLy1 indicates lymphangitis is present and confined to the area around the primary tumour, cLy2 indicated lymphangitis at a distance from the primary tumour but confined to the lobe of the primary, cLy3 indicates lymphangitis in other ipsilateral lobes and cLy4 indicates lymphangitis affecting the contralateral lung. Radiologists and clinicians are encouraged to collect this information for future analysis.

f) All cases in which there is metastatic spread to distant organs are classified as M1b if there is a single metastasis or M1c if there are multiple extrathoracic metastasis in one or in several organs. However, there are clear differences in prognosis based upon tumour burden and the critical nature of some organ sites. Such differences will influence the choice of treatment and the intent of treatment by all modalities of care. Selected patients with isolated metastases to a single organ may benefit from surgical treatment. Clinicians, oncologists and surgeons are encouraged to fully document the extent of disease in M1b and M1c cases, collecting data on all of the sites of (suspected) metastatic disease and whether such organs contain single or multiple deposits.

g) The designation of additional tumour nodules of similar histological appearance in the lung(s) were re-classified in the 7th edition of TNM[6] and were kept unchanged in the 8th edition.[7] The UICC cannot determine that this is valid for cases in which multiple deposits are encountered and prospective data collection is necessary to fully validate this re-classification. It is recommended that radiologists, oncologists, surgeons and pathologists document in their clinical and pathological staging the number of nodules in the lobe of the primary, other ipsilateral lobes and the contralateral lung and the diameter of the largest deposit in each location. When found in the lobe of the primary, T3 disease, the size of the closest nodule from the primary tumour and its distance from the primary tumour should also be documented.

h) Carcinoid tumours are included within the 7th and 8th editions of TNM. This validates its use by surgeons and pathologists over several decades. However, further details are needed to assess the prognostic impact of certain features in carcinoid tumours:[8] typical versus atypical features, T size cut points, the prognostic impact of multiple deposits and whether these are associated with the syndrome of Diffuse Idiopathic Neuroendocrine Cell Hyperplasia (DIPNECH). In addition, in carcinoid tumours, in which long-term survival can be expected even when associated with multiple tumour nodules or nodal disease, it is important to collect data on disease specific survival. Clinicians, oncologists, surgeons and pathologists are urged to collect such data prospectively.

i) PET scanning using FDG is now widely utilized and has had an impact of the accuracy of clinical staging and referrals for surgical treatment. In addition, a meta-analysis has shown that PET features, such as the maximum value of the Standardized Uptake Value (SUVmax) in the primary tumour prior to treatment is an independent prognostic factor.[9] Nuclear medicine specialists, clinicians and oncologists are encouraged to document the use of PET in clinical staging of lung cancer, and to record features such as SUV(max) in the primary and any nodal and/or metastatic sites.

References

1. Rami-Porta R, Wittekind C, Goldstraw P. Complete resection in lung cancer surgery:proposed definition. *Lung Cancer* 2005; 49: 25-33.
2. Lim E, Clough R, Goldstraw P et al. Impact of positive pleural lavage cytology on survival of patients having lung resection for non-small-cell lung cancer: An international individual patient data meta-analysis. *J Thorac Cardiovasc Surg* 2010; 139: 1441-1446.
3. Travis WD, Brambilla E, Rami-Porta R, et al. Visceral pleural invasion: Pathologic criteria and use of elastic stains: Proposals for the 7th edition of the TNM classification for lung cancer. *J Thorac Oncol* 2008; 3: 1384-1390.
4. The Japan Lung Cancer Society. Classification of Lung Cancer: First English Edition. 1 ed. Chiba: Kanehara and Co; 2000.
5. Hammar SP. Common Tumors. In: Dail DH, Hammar SP, editors. Pulmonary Pathology. 2nd ed. New York: Springer-Verlag; 1994. p. 1138.
6. Rami-Porta R, Ball D, Crowley JJ, et al. The IASLC Lung Cancer Staging Project: proposals for the revision of the T descriptors in the forthcoming (seventh) edition of the TNM classification for lung cancer. *J Thorac Oncol* 2007; 2: 593-602.

7. Rami-Porta R, Bolejack V, Crowley J et al. The IASLC lung cancer staging project: proposals for the revisions of the T descriptors in the forthcoming 8th edition of the TNM classification for lung cancer. *J Thorac Oncol* 2015; 10: 990-1003.

8. Travis WD, Giroux DJ, Chansky K, et al. The IASLC Lung Cancer Staging Project: proposals for the inclusion of bronchopulmonary carcinoid tumours in the forthcoming (seventh) edition of the TNM classification for lung cancer. *J Thorac Oncol* 2008; 3:1213-1223.

9. Berghmans T, Dusart M, Paesmans M, et al. Primary tumour standardized uptake value (SUV max) measured on florodeoxyglucose emission tomography (PDG-PET) is of prognostic value for survival in non-small cell lung cancer (NSCLC): A systematic review and meta-analysis (MA) by the European Lung Cancer Working Party for the IASLC Lung Cancer Staging Project. *J Thorac Oncol* 2008; 3: 6-12.

8

New Site-Specific Recommendations Proposed by the IASLC

Ramón Rami-Porta, Frank C. Detterbeck, William D. Travis, and Hisao Asamura

The following recommendations for lung cancer classification derive from the analyses of the International Association for the Study of Lung Cancer (IASLC) database, the review of published articles, and a wide international and multidisciplinary consensus. The new categories for adenocarcinoma *in situ* and minimally invasive adenocarcinoma have been accepted by the Union for International Cancer Control (UICC) and by the American Joint Committee on Cancer (AJCC), and will appear in the 8th edition of their respective staging manuals; the other recommendations are included in the 8th edition of the AJCC *Cancer Staging Manual*, but are still under assessment by the UICC. Presumably, they will appear in the 5th edition of the UICC *TNM Supplement – A Commentary on Uniform Use* that is traditionally published after the UICC *TNM Classification of Malignant Tumours*.

New Categories for the New Adenocarcinomas

Adenocarcinoma *in situ* is classified as Tis (AIS) to differentiate it from squamous cell carcinoma *in situ*, which is classified as Tis (SCIS).[1] Tis (AIS) and Tis (SCIS) N0 M0 are stage 0.[2]

Minimally invasive adenocarcinoma is classified as T1mi.[1] T1mi N0 M0 is stage IA1, together with T1a N0 M0.[2]

Measurement of Tumour Size in Part-Solid Non-Mucinous Adenocarcinomas

Part-solid adenocarcinomas present with a solid component and a ground glass opacity on computed tomography (CT). At pathological examination, the solid component usually corresponds to the invasive part; and the ground glass opacity, to the lepidic part. To define the T category by tumour size, only the size of the solid component on CT or the size of the invasive component at pathologic examination are considered, because it is the size of the solid/invasive component that determines prognosis. However, documentation of both the size of the solid component/invasive part and of the whole tumour including the ground glass and lepidic components in radiology and pathology reports, respectively, is recommended.[1]

Measurement of Tumour Size after Induction Therapy

This issue has been rarely discussed in depth before. The recommendation of the IASLC is that tumour size can be measured by multiplying the percentage of viable tumour cells by the total size of the tumour.[1]

Classification of Lung Cancers with Multiple Sites of Involvement

To avoid ambiguity and to facilitate the homogeneous classification of lung cancer with multiple sites of disease, an *ad hoc* sub-committee of the IASLC Staging and Prognostic Factors Committee developed the following recommendations based on the analyses of the IASLC database where data were available, the review of published reports and a wide multidisciplinary and international consensus. The following recommendations apply to grossly identified tumours and to those identified at microscopic examination, and differ depending on the pattern of disease.[3]

- **Synchronous and metachronous primary lung cancers.** Regardless of tumour location, a separate TNM is defined for each tumour. The clinical and pathological criteria to differentiate second primary from related tumours are defined in Table 8.1.[4]
- **Separate tumour nodules with similar histopathologic features (intrapulmonary metastases).** Classification depends on the location of the separate tumour nodule(s): T3 if the separate tumour nodule(s) is(are) in the same lobe of the primary tumour; T4, if located in a different ipsilateral lobe; M1a, if located in the contralateral lung. If there are additional extrathoracic metastases, the tumour will be classified as M1b or M1c depending on the number of metastatic sites. The clinical and pathological criteria to categorise separate tumour nodules (intrathoracic metastasis) are defined in Table 8.2.[5]
- **Multifocal pulmonary adenocarcinoma with ground glass/lepidic features.** Regardless of the location of the tumours, the rule of the highest T with the number (#) or (m) for multiple in parentheses, and an N and an M for all of the multiple tumours collectively applies for these tumours. Table 8.3 shows the clinical and pathologic criteria to define these tumours.[6]
- **Diffuse pneumonic-type lung adenocarcinoma.** A) Single focus of disease. The general TNM classification is applied, with the T category defined by tumour size. B) Multiple foci of disease. Tumour classification is based on the location

Table 8.1. Criteria for separate versus related pulmonary tumours.[4]

Clinical Criteria*

Tumours may be considered separate primary tumours if:
They are clearly of a different histologic type (e.g. squamous carcinoma and adenocarcinoma) by biopsy

Tumours may be considered to be arising from a single tumour source if:
Exactly matching breakpoints are identified by comparative genomic hybridization

Relative arguments that favor separate tumours:
Different radiographic appearance or metabolic uptake
Different biomarker pattern (driver gene mutations)
Different rates of growth (if previous imaging is available)
Absence of nodal or systemic metastases

Relative arguments that favor a single tumour source:
Same radiographic appearance
Similar growth patterns (if previous imaging is available)
Significant nodal or systemic metastases
Same biomarker pattern (and same histotype)

Pathologic Criteria (i.e. after resection)**

Tumours may be considered separate primary tumours if:
They are clearly of a different histologic type (e.g. squamous carcinoma and adenocarcinoma)
They are clearly different by a comprehensive histologic assessment
They are squamous carcinomas that have arisen from carcinoma in situ

Tumours may be considered to be arising from a single tumour source if:
Exactly matching breakpoints are identified by comparative genomic hybridization

Relative arguments that favor separate tumours (to be considered together with clinical factors):
Different pattern of biomarkers
Absence of nodal or systemic metastases

Relative arguments that favor a single tumour source (to be considered together with clinical factors):
Matching appearance on comprehensive histologic assessment
Same biomarker pattern
Significant nodal or systemic metastases

*Note that a comprehensive histologic assessment is not included in clinical staging, as it requires that the entire specimen has been resected.
**Pathologic information should be supplemented with any clinical information that is available.

Table 8.2. Criteria to categorize a lesion as a separate tumour nodule (intrapulmonary metastasis).[3,5]

Clinical Criteria

Tumours should be considered to have a separate tumour nodule(s) if:
There is a solid lung cancer and a separate tumour nodule(s) with a similar solid appearance and with (presumed) matching histologic appearance
- This applies whether or not a biopsy has been performed on the lesions, provided that there is strong suspicion that the lesions are histologically identical
- This applies whether or not there are sites of extrathoracic metastases

AND provided that:
The lesions are NOT judged to be synchronous primary lung cancers

The lesions are NOT multifocal GG/L lung cancer (multiple nodules with ground glass/lepidic features) or pneumonic-type of lung cancer

Pathologic Criteria

Tumours should be considered to have a separate tumour nodule(s) (intrapulmonary metastasis) if:
There is a separate tumour nodule(s) of cancer in the lung with a similar histologic appearance to a primary lung cancer

AND provided that:
The lesions are NOT judged to be synchronous primary lung cancers
The lesions are NOT multiple foci of LPA, MIA, AIS

Note: a radiographically solid appearance and the specific histologic subtype of solid adenocarcinoma denote different things.

AIS, adenocarcinoma in situ; GG/L, ground glass/lepidic; LPA, lepidic predominant adenocarcinoma; MIA, minimally invasive adenocarcinoma

of the involved areas (including miliary involvement): T3, if located in one lobe; T4, if located in other ipsilateral lobes; M1a, if the contralateral lung is involved, with the T category defined by the largest tumour. C) If tumour size is difficult to determine: T4 applies if there is evidence of involvement of another ipsilateral lobe. In all circumstances, the N category should apply to all pulmonary sites and the appropriate M category should be applied depending on the number and location of metastases. The clinical and pathological criteria to define these tumours are shown in Table 8.4.[6]

The basic radiographic and pathologic features, the recommended TNM classification and the conceptual view of the four patterns of lung cancer with multiple sites of involvement are summarised in Table 8.5.

Table 8.3. Criteria identifying multifocal ground glass/lepidic lung adenocarcinoma.[6]

Clinical Criteria

Tumours should be considered multifocal GG/L lung adenocarcinoma if:
There are multiple sub-solid nodules (either pure ground glass or part-solid), with at least one suspected (or proven) to be cancer

- This applies whether or not a biopsy has been performed of the nodules

- This applies if the other nodules(s) are found on biopsy to be AIS, MIA or LPA

- This applies if a nodule has become >50% solid but is judged to have arisen from a GGN, provided there are other sub-solid nodules

- GGN lesions <5mm or lesions suspected to be AAH are not counted

Pathologic Criteria

Tumours should be considered multifocal GG/L lung adenocarcinoma if:
There are multiple foci of LPA, MIA, or AIS

- This applies whether a detailed histologic assessment (i.e. proportion of subtypes, etc.) shows a matching or different appearance

- This applies if one lesion(s) is LPA, MIA or AIS and there are other sub-solid nodules of which a biopsy has not been performed.

- This applies whether the nodule(s) are identified preoperatively or only on pathologic examination

- Foci of AAH are not counted

Note: a radiographically solid appearance and the specific histologic subtype of solid adenocarcinoma denote different things.

AIS, adenocarcinoma in situ; GG/L, ground glass/lepidic; LPA, lepidic predominant adenocarcinoma; MIA, minimally invasive adenocarcinoma

Quantification of Nodal Disease

Quantification of nodal disease has prognostic impact. For the 7th edition of the TNM classification of lung cancer, quantification of nodal disease was based on the number of involved nodal zones.[7] For the 8th edition, it is based on the number of involved nodal stations.[8] Both criteria separate groups of tumours with statistically significant differences. However, both were based on pathological findings of the lymphadenectomy specimen that could not be validated at clinical staging. The recommendation from the IASLC is to quantify nodal disease at pathological staging because it allows the refinement of postoperative prognosis and assists in making decisions on adjuvant therapy, but also to try to quantify it at clinical staging with the available means. The subclassification of nodal disease based on the number of involved nodal stations is as follows:

- N1a: single station N1
- N1b: multiple station N1
- N2a1: single station N2 without N1 disease (skip metastasis)

Table 8.4. Criteria identifying the pneumonic-type of adenocarcinoma.[6]

Clinical Criteria

Tumours should be considered pneumonic-type of adenocarcinoma if:
The cancer manifests in a regional distribution, similar to a pneumonic infiltrate or consolidation

- This applies whether there is one confluent area or multiple regions of disease. The region(s) may be confined to one lobe, in multiple lobes, or bilateral, but should involve a regional pattern of distribution.
- The involved areas may appear to be ground glass, solid consolidation or a combination thereof.
- This can be applied when there is compelling suspicion of malignancy whether or not a biopsy has been performed of the area(s).
- This should not be applied to discrete nodules (i.e. GG/L nodules)
- This should not be applied to tumours causing bronchial obstruction with resultant obstructive pneumonia or atelectasis

Pathologic Criteria

Tumours should be considered pneumonic-type of adenocarcinoma if:
There is diffuse distribution of adenocarcinoma throughout a region(s) of the lung, as opposed to a single well-demarcated mass or multiple discrete well-demarcated nodules

- This typically involves an invasive mucinous adenocarcinoma, although a mixed mucinous and non-mucinous pattern may occur.
- The tumour may show a heterogeneous mixture of acinar, papillary and micropapillary growth patterns, although it is usually lepidic predominant.

Note: a radiographically solid appearance and the specific histologic subtype of solid adenocarcinoma denote different things.

GG/L, ground glass/lepidic

- N2a2: single station N2 with N1 disease
- N2b: multiple station N2

Prognosis worsens as the number of involved nodal stations increases, but N1b and N2a1 have the same prognosis.[8]

References

1. Travis WD, Asamura H, Bankier A et al. The IASLC Lung Cancer Staging Project: proposals for coding T categories for subsolid nodules and assessment of tumor size in part-solid tumors in the forthcoming eighth edition of the TNM classification of lung cancer. *J Thorac Oncol* 2016; 11: 1204-1223.
2. Goldstraw P, Chansky K, Crowley J et al. The IASLC Lung Cancer Staging Project: proposals for the revision of the stage grouping in the forthcoming (8th) edition of the TNM classification of lung cancer. *J Thorac Oncol* 2016; 11: 39-51.
3. Detterbeck FC, Nicholson AG, Franklin WA et al. The IASLC Lung Cancer Staging Project: summary of proposals for revisions of the classification of lung cancers with multiple pulmonary sites of involvement in the forthcoming eighth edition of the TNM classification. *J Thorac Oncol* 2016; 11: 539-650.

Table 8.5. Schematic summary of patterns of disease and TNM classification of patients with lung cancer with multiple pulmonary sites of involvement.[3]

	Second Primary Lung Cancer	Separate Tumour Nodule (Intrapulmonary metastasis)	Multifocal GG/L Nodules	Pneumonic-Type of Adenocarcinoma
Imaging features	Two or more distinct masses with imaging characteristics of lung cancer (e.g. spiculated)	Typical lung cancer (e.g. solid, spiculated) with separate solid nodule	Multiple ground glass or part-solid nodules	Patchy areas of ground glass and consolidation
Pathologic features	Different histotype or different morphology by comprehensive histologic assessment	Distinct masses with the same morphologic features by comprehensive histologic assessment	Adenocarcinomas with prominent lepidic component (typically varying degrees of AIS, MIA, LPA)	Same histologic features throughout (most often invasive mucinous adenocarcinoma)
TNM classification	Separate cTNM and pTNM for each cancer	Location of separate nodule relative to primary site determines if T3, T4 or M1a; single N and M	T based on highest T lesion with (#/m) indicating multiplicity; single N and M	T based on size or T3 if in single lobe, T4 or M1a if in different ipsilateral or contralateral lobes; single N and M
Conceptual view	Unrelated tumours	Single tumour, with intrapulmonary metastasis	Separate tumours, albeit with similarities	Single tumour, diffuse pulmonary involvement

AIS, adenocarcinoma in situ; GG/L, ground glass/lepidic; LPA, lepidic-predominant adenocarcinoma; MIA, minimally invasive adenocarcinoma; p, pathologic; TNM, tumour, node, metastasis.

4. Detterbeck FC, Franklin WA, Nicholson AG et al. The IASLC Lung Cancer Staging Project: background data and proposed criteria to distinguish separate primary lung cancers from metastatic foci in patients with two lung tumors in the forthcoming eighth edition of the TNM classification for lung cancer. *J Thorac Oncol* 2016; 11: 651-665.
5. Detterbeck FC, Bolejack V, Arenberg DA et al. The IASLC Lung Cancer Staging Project: background data and proposals for the classification of lung cancer with separate tumor nodules in the forthcoming eighth edition of the TNM classification for lung cancer. *J Thorac Oncol* 2016; 11: 681-692.
6. Detterbeck FC, Marom EM, Arenberg DA et al. The IASLC Lung Cancer Staging Project: background data and proposals for the application of TNM staging rules to lung cancer presenting as multiple nodules with ground glass or lepidic features or a pneumonic-type of involvement in the forthcoming eighth edition of the TNM classification. *J Thorac Oncol* 2016; 11: 666-680.

7. Rusch VW, Crowley J, Giroux DJ, et al. The IASLC Lung Cancer Staging Project: proposals for the revision of the N descriptors in the forthcoming seventh edition of the TNM classifications for lung cancer. *J Thorac Oncol* 2007; 2: 603-612.

8. Asamura H, Chansky K, Crowley J et al. The IASLC Lung Cancer Staging Project: proposals for the revisions of the N descriptors in the forthcoming 8th edition of the TNM classification for lung cancer. *J Thorac Oncol* 2015; 10: 1675-1684.

9

Atlas of Lung Cancer Staging

T1a, T1b   **T1c**

Tumour:
≤1cm

Tumour:
>2cm, ≤3cm

Tumour:
>1cm,
≤2cm

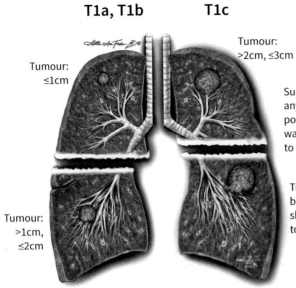

Superficial spreading tumour of any size with its invasive component limited to the bronchial wall, which may extend proximal to the main bronchus is T1

Tumour ≤3cm; any associated bronchoscopic invasion should not extend proximal to the lobar bronchus

T2a   **T2b**

Tumour:
> 3cm, ≤ 4cm

Tumour ≤ 4cm, invasion of the visceral pleura

Tumour involves main bronchus, regardless of distance from carina but without carinal involvement

Associated atelectasis or obstructive pneumonitis that extends to the hilar region, either involving part of the lung or the entire lung

Tumour in the main bronchus < 2cm from the carina (without involvement of the carina) and/or associated atelectasis or obstructive pneumonitis of the entire lung

Tumour:
> 4cm, ≤ 5cm
(with or without other T2 descriptors)

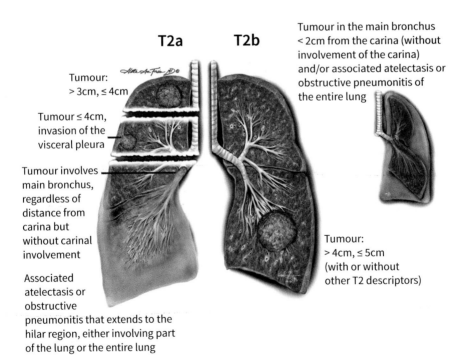

Note: if the tumour is associated with atelectasis or pneumonitis, it is T2a if lesion ≤ 4cm or if tumour size cannot be measured; it is T2b if lesion > 4cm, ≤ 5cm.

T3

Chest wall invasion, including Pancoast tumours without invasion of vertebral body or spinal canal, encasement of the subclavian vessels, or unequivocal involvement of the superior branches of the brachial plexus (C8 or above)

Tumour:
> 5cm, ≤ 7cm

Invasion of parietal pleura

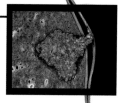

Phrenic nerve or parietal pericardium invasion

Separate tumour nodule(s) in the lobe of the primary

T4

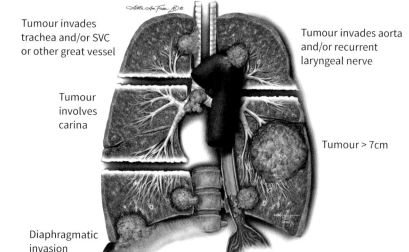

Tumour invades trachea and/or SVC or other great vessel

Tumour invades aorta and/or recurrent laryngeal nerve

Tumour involves carina

Tumour > 7cm

Diaphragmatic invasion

Tumour invades adjacent vertebral body

Tumour invades oesophagus, mediastinum and/or heart

Pancoast tumours with invasion of one or more of the following structures:
- vertebral body or spinal canal
- brachial plexus (C8 or above)
- subclavian vessels

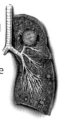

Tumour accompanied by ipsilateral, separate tumour nodules, different lobe

N0

N1

No regional
lymph node
metastases

Metastasis
in ipsilateral
intrapulmonary/
peribronchial/
hilar lymph node(s),
including nodal
involvement by
direct extension

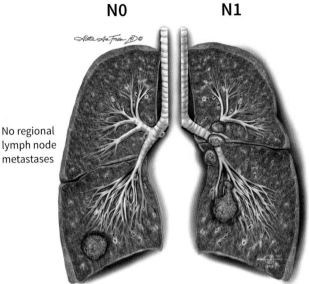

N2

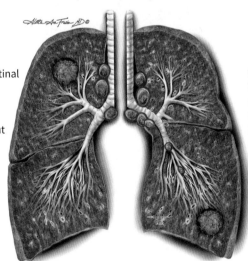

Metastasis in
ipsilateral mediastinal
and/or subcarinal
lymph node(s),
including "skip"
metastasis without
N1 involvement

Metastasis in
ipsilateral
mediastinal
and/or subcarinal
lymph node(s)
associated with
N1 disease

N3

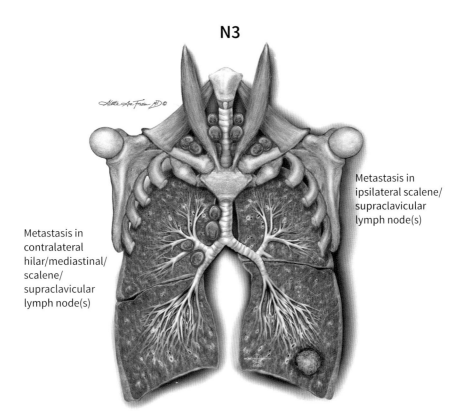

Metastasis in
contralateral
hilar/mediastinal/
scalene/
supraclavicular
lymph node(s)

Metastasis in
ipsilateral scalene/
supraclavicular
lymph node(s)

M1a

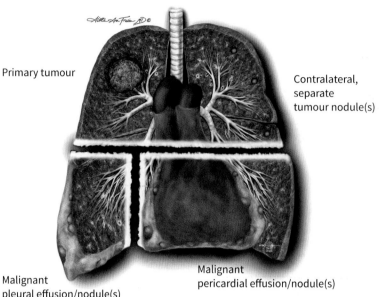

Primary tumour

Contralateral,
separate
tumour nodule(s)

Malignant
pleural effusion/nodule(s)

Malignant
pericardial effusion/nodule(s)

Note: when the pleural (pericardial)
effusions are negative after multiple
microscopic examinations, and the fluid
is non-bloody and not an exudate, they
should be excluded as a staging descriptor.

M1b

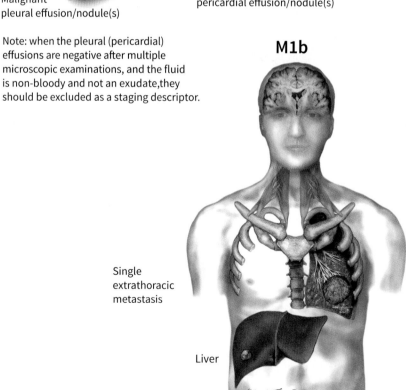

Single
extrathoracic
metastasis

Liver

M1b

This includes involvement of a single distant (non-regional) lymph node

M1c

Brain

Lymph nodes

Bone

This includes multiple extrathoracic metastases in one or several organs

Liver

Adrenal

PART III

PLEURAL MESOTHELIOMA

10

The History of TNM Staging in Malignant Pleural Mesothelioma

Valerie W. Rusch, Dorothy Giroux, and Harvey I. Pass

Early MPM Staging Systems

During the past 40 years, several staging systems for malignant pleural mesothelioma (MPM) were proposed. Prior to the International Mesothelioma Interest Group (IMIG) Staging System[1], earlier systems were imprecise and not evidence-based. A classification proposed by Butchart was a simple stage-based rather than a tumour, node, and metastasis (TNM) system. The extent of lymph node involvement and chest wall invasion was poorly described.[2] Mattson's classification defined contralateral tumour involvement as stage II rather than stage III and has been abandoned.[3] Chahinian was the first to devise a TNM-based MPM staging system that considered parameters such as locoregional lymph node involvement and specific sites and extent of tumour invasion.[4]

Origins of the International Mesothelioma Interest Group (IMIG) Staging System

In 1994, at a workshop co-sponsored by the IASLC and IMIG, MPM investigators analyzed published surgical databases and the available small clinical trials in this disease. The data were used to create a TNM-based system that could be applied to the clinical and pathologic staging of MPM.[5] One of the important features of the IMIG Staging System was that, guided by the work of Boutin,[6] it separated out patients with early tumours according to the extent and depth of pleural involvement. The IMIG staging system was accepted by the Union for International Cancer Control (UICC) and the American Joint Committee on Cancer (AJCC) as the first international MPM staging system for the 6th and 7th editions of their staging manuals. Shortly after it was adopted by the AJCC and UICC, the IMIG staging system was validated in two surgical series of MPM, and thereafter was widely used in retrospective analyses and prospective clinical trials.[1,7]

Nevertheless, there was concern about the validity of the IMIG staging system because it was derived primarily from small, retrospective surgical series, and was difficult to apply to clinical staging in patients not managed surgically. Also, the nodal (N) component of this system was not evidence-based and was simply adopted from that used for lung cancer. In 1999, Sugargaker et al. proposed the alternative Brigham Staging System based on tumour, resectability and nodal status.[8] However, this was also a surgically based classification that included factors other than the anatomic extent of disease. In 2010, a single institution re-evaluation of the Brigham System was published which examined pathologic characteristics and explored correlations with outcome among 354 patients with epithelioid MPM who underwent extrapleural pneumonectomy (EPP).[9] T classification criteria were adjusted based on margin status (negative for T1) and were only minimally concordant with the IMIG system with regard to the classification of T4. Internal mammary or inferior mediastinal nodal station involvement were grouped in Stage I since these were associated with significantly longer overall survival relative to involved lymph nodes in the superior mediastinum (which were grouped as Stages II, III or IV). These analyses raised the issue of whether patients undergoing surgical resections other than EPP and patients with non-epithelioid tumour histology should be staged separately. It was clear that a large international staging database was needed to inform changes to the staging system in this rare disease.

The First IASLC MPM Database

In an effort modeled on the revisions that the IASLC proposed for lung cancer staging for the 7th editions of the UICC and AJCC manuals, the IASLC, in collaboration with members of the IMIG, developed a large international database. Data were initially solicited from surgeons around the world known to care for a high volume of MPM patients and were transmitted to the statistical center, Cancer Research And Biostatistics (CRAB) in Seattle, Washington. Common data elements were established after review of each institutional database and the time frame chosen for data was 1995 to 2009. The project was initiated in 2009 at IASLC Workshop on Advances in Mesothelioma, at which time a "white paper" detailing uniform definitions for the use of surgery in mesothelioma was also planned in order to standardize the description of surgical cytoreductive procedures. Since the "white paper" was being formulated in parallel with the retrospective registry, the surgical procedures in the original database were classified simply as operations performed with either palliative or curative intent. The former included exploration, no resection, and palliative (i.e., partial) pleurectomy whereas the latter included extrapleural pneumonectomy (EPP), pleurectomy/decortication (P/D) for resection of all gross tumours, and P/D combined with anatomical lung resection other than pneumonectomy. Data were submitted on 3,101 patients from 15 centers on 4 continents, with publication in 2012.[10] Because both clinical (cTNM) and pathological (pTNM) staging data were not available on all patients, cTNM and pTNM staging information were combined in 2,316 patients to provide "best" staging (bTNM) in accordance with AJCC and UICC guidelines. Most patients (64.5%) had curative intent procedures with approximately half undergoing EPP. Although overall survival data largely supported continued use of the original IMIG staging system, several important areas for improvement were identified. Key findings of the analyses were that (1) there was *poor* correlation between cTNM and pTNM staging, especially for clinical stages I and II, emphasizing the need for improvement in methods of clinical staging; (2) the stage groupings effectively separated patients by their median survival, but far more detailed data were needed to revise the T and N categories; (3) epithelioid histology was associated with the best outcome and sarcomatoid, the worst; (4) survival was significantly influenced by whether the surgical procedure was performed with curative versus palliative intent (median survival 18 versus 12 months) and by the use of adjuvant therapy; (5) stage I tumours resected by EPP for curative intent were associated with a median survival of 40 months while those managed by P/D, supposedly for curative intent, had a median survival of 23 months, but no differences in survival between EPP and P/D were identified in patients with higher stage disease. Multivariable analyses identified factors independently influencing survival including overall tumour stage, T category, N category, tumour histology, patient sex, age, and type of operation. However, there was no significant survival difference between stages I and II, highlighting the need to revise these stage categories.

The "white paper," published in 2011, was a premeditated strategy in order to deal with cytoreductive classification issues for the future.[11] Procedure-based definitions resulted from a web-based survey of 62 experienced MPM surgeons from 39 medical centers in 14 countries. The "white paper" led the International Staging Committee of the IASLC to recommend that EPP describe complete gross tumour resection via removal of the entire pleura and lung with or without excision of the pericardium and diaphragm, and that P/D describe removal of all macroscopic tumour involving the parietal and visceral pleura and that the term "extended" P/D (or EPD) be used to describe parietal and visceral pleurectomy in conjunction with resection of the diaphragm and/or pericardium.

Analyses of Supplementary Prognostic Variables in the First IASLC MPM Database

There was information in the database on supplementary clinical variables for MPM that included the use of chemotherapy or radiotherapy at any time (adjuvant therapy), smoking history, history of asbestos exposure, history of weight loss (defined as greater than 5% versus less than 5% in the previous 6 months), Eastern Cooperative Oncology Group (ECOG) performance status, chest pain, and dyspnoea. Laboratory parameters included haemoglobin, white blood cell count, and platelet count. A total of 2141 patients with best tumour, node, metastasis (TNM) stages (pathologic with/without clinical staging) could be used to develop prognostic models for three scenarios including the patient having cytoreductive surgery (Scenario A), the individual with only clinical TNM (Scenario B), and the newly diagnosed patient with limited data (Scenario C).[12] These prognostic models were defined as follows: **Scenario A:** best pathologic stage, histology, sex, age, type of surgery, adjuvant treatment, white blood cell count (WBC) (≥15.5 or not), and platelets (≥400 k or not) (n=550). **Scenario B:** clinical stage, histology, sex, age, type of surgery, adjuvant treatment, WBC, haemoglobin (<14.6 or not), and platelets (n=627). **Scenario C:** histology, sex, age, WBC, haemoglobin, and platelets (n=906).

The Second IASLC MPM Database

To plan for the 8th editions of the AJCC and UICC staging systems, a new IASLC MPM database was created that would address controversies raised by the initial analysis. Initiated in July 2013, this second IASLC MPM database included more granular information regarding T, N and M descriptors and an electronic data capture (EDC) system developed at CRAB. Additional investigators who could provide valid information on patients staged clinically and managed non-surgically were recruited. As of the closure for data submission in June 2014, a total of 3,519 MPM cases were entered from 29 centers spanning 4 continents, of which 2,460 were considered eligible for analysis after data review. Cases diagnosed as early as 1995 were included provided that they met data quality standards, but most were diagnosed between 2000 and 2013. Cases diagnosed after June 30, 3013 were excluded and analyses were undertaken in the end of 2014, allowing a minimum potential follow-up of 18 months. Analyses of this second IASLC database now form the basis for revision of the TNM categories and stage groupings in the 8th editions of the AJCC and UICC MPM staging systems.

References

1. Rusch VW, Venkatraman E. The importance of surgical staging in the treatment of malignant pleural mesothelioma. *J Thorac Cardiovasc Surg* 1996;111:815-26.
2. Butchart EG, Ashcroft T, Barnsley WC, Holden MP. Pleuropneumonectomy in the management of diffuse malignant mesothelioma of the pleura. Experience with 29 patients. *Thorax* 1976;31:15-24.
3. Tammilehto L, Kivisaari L, Salminen US, Maasilta P, Mattson K. Evaluation of the clinical TNM staging system for malignant pleural mesothelioma: An assessment in 88 patients. *Lung Cancer* 1995;12: 25-34.
4. Chahinian AP. Therapeutic modalities in malignant pleural mesothelioma. In: Chretien J, Hirsch A, editors. Diseases of the Pleura. New York: Masson; 1983, p. 224-36.

5. Rusch VW, The International Mesothelioma Interest Group. A proposed new international TNM staging system for malignant pleural mesothelioma. *Chest* 1995;108:1122-8.

6. Boutin C, Rey F, Gouvernet J, Viallat J-R, Astoul P, Ledoray V. Thoracoscopy in pleural malignant mesothelioma: A prospective study of 188 consecutive patients. Part 2: Prognosis and staging. *Cancer* 1993;72:394-404.

7. Pass HI, Temeck BK, Kranda K, Steinberg SM, Feuerstein IR. Preoperative tumor volume is associated with outcome in malignant pleural mesothelioma. *J Thorac Cardiovasc Surg* 1998;115:310-8.

8. Sugarbaker DJ, Flores RM, Jaklitsch MT, et al. Resection margins, extrapleural nodal status, and cell type determine postoperative long-term survival in trimodality therapy of malignant pleural mesothelioma: Results of 183 patients. *J Thorac Cardiovasc Surg* 1999;117:54-65.

9. Richards WG, Godleski JJ, Yeap BY, et al. Proposed adjustments to pathologic staging of epithelial malignant pleural mesothelioma based on analysis of 354 cases. *Cancer* 2010;116:1510-7.

10. Rusch VW, Giroux D, Kennedy C, et al. Initial analysis of the International Association for the Study of Lung Cancer Mesothelioma Database. *J Thorac Oncol* 2012;7:1631-9.

11. Rice D, Rusch V, Pass H, et al. Recommendations for uniform definitions of surgical techniques for malignant pleural mesothelioma: A consensus report of the International Association for the Study of Lung Cancer International Staging Committee and the International Mesothelioma Interest Group. *J Thorac Oncol* 2011;6(8):1304-12.

12. Pass HI, Giroux D, Kennedy C, et al. Supplementary prognostic variables for pleural mesothelioma: A report from the IASLC Staging Committee. *J Thorac Oncol* 2014;9(6): 856-64.

Acknowledgment: Used with the permission of the Union for International Cancer Control (UICC), Geneva, Switzerland. The original source for this material is in Brierley JB, Gospodarowicz MK, Wittekind Ch, eds. UICC TNM Classification of Malignant Tumours, 8th edition (2017), published by John Wiley & Sons, Ltd, www.wiley.com.

11

8th Edition of TNM for Pleural Mesothelioma

Introductory Notes

The classification applies to malignant mesothelioma of pleura.
Each site is described under the following headings:

- Rules for classification with the procedures for assessing T, N, and M categories; additional methods may be used when they enhance the accuracy of appraisal before treatment
- Anatomical subsites where appropriate
- Definition of the regional lymph nodes
- TNM clinical classification
- pTNM pathological classification
- Stage
- Prognostic factors grid

Regional Lymph Nodes

The regional lymph nodes extend from the supraclavicular region to the diaphragm. Direct extension of the primary tumour into lymph nodes is classified as lymph node metastasis.

Pleural Mesothelioma
(ICD-O C38.4)

Rules for Classification

The classification applies only to malignant mesothelioma of the pleura.
There should be histological confirmation of the disease.
   Changes in this edition from the seventh edition are based upon recommen-

dations from the International Association for the Study of Lung Cancer (IASLC) Staging Project.[1-5]

The following are the procedures for assessing T, N, and M categories:

T categories   Physical examination, imaging, endoscopy, and/or surgical exploration

N categories   Physical examination, imaging, endoscopy, and/or surgical exploration

M categories   Physical examination, imaging, and/or surgical exploration

Regional Lymph Nodes

The regional lymph nodes are the intrathoracic, internal mammary, scalene, and supraclavicular nodes.

TNM Clinical Classification

T – Primary Tumour

TX   Primary tumour cannot be assessed.

T0   No evidence of primary tumour

T1   Tumour involves ipsilateral parietal or visceral pleura only, with or without involvement of visceral, mediastinal or diaphragmatic pleura.

T2   Tumour involves the ipsilateral pleura (parietal or visceral pleura), with at least one of the following:
  • invasion of diaphragmatic muscle
  • invasion of lung parenchyma

T3   Tumour involves ipsilateral pleura (parietal or visceral pleura), with at least one of the following:
  • invasion of endothoracic fascia
  • invasion into mediastinal fat
  • solitary focus of tumour invading soft tissues of the chest wall
  • non-transmural involvement of the pericardium

T4   Tumour involves ipsilateral pleura (parietal or visceral pleura), with at least one of the following:
  • chest wall, with or without associated rib destruction (diffuse or multifocal)
  • peritoneum (via direct transdiaphragmatic extension)
  • contralateral pleura
  • mediastinal organs (oesophagus, trachea, heart, great vessels)
  • vertebra, neuroforamen, spinal cord
  • internal surface of the pericardium (transmural invasion with or without a pericardial effusion)

N – Regional Lymph Nodes

NX   Regional lymph nodes cannot be assessed

N0   No regional lymph node metastasis

N1   Metastases to ipsilateral intrathoracic lymph nodes (includes ipsilateral bronchopulmonary, hilar, subcarinal, paratracheal, aortopulmonary, para-esophageal, peridiaphragmatic, pericardial fat pad, intercostal and internal mammary nodes)

N2   Metastases to contralateral intrathoracic lymph nodes. Metastases to ipsilateral or contralateral supraclavicular lymph nodes

M – Distant Metastasis

M0   No distant metastasis

M1   Distant metastasis

pTNM Pathological Classification

The pT and pN categories correspond to the T and N categories. For pM see page 59.

Stage – Pleural Mesothelioma

Stage IA	T1	N0	M0
Stage IB	T2, T3	N0	M0
Stage II	T1, T2	N1	M0
Stage IIIA	T3	N1	M0
Stage IIIB	T1. T2, T3	N2	M0
	T4	Any N	M0
Stage IV	Any T	Any N	M1

References

1. Rusch VW, Giroux D, Kennedy C et al. Initial analysis of the International Association for the Study of Lung Cancer Mesothelioma database. *J Thorac Oncol* 2012; 7: 1631-1639.
2. Pass H, Giroux D, Kennedy C et al. The IASLC Mesothelioma database: improving staging of a rare disease through international participation. *J Thorac Oncol* 2016; in press.
3. Nowak AK, Chansky K, Rice DC et al. The IASLC Mesothelioma Staging Project: proposals for revisions of the T descriptors in the forthcoming eighth edition of the TNM classification for mesothelioma. *J Thorac Oncol* 2016; in press.
4. Rice D, Chansky K, Nowak A et al. The IASLC Mesothelioma Staging Project: proposals for revisions of the N descriptors in the forthcoming eighth edition of the TNM classification for malignant pleural mesothelioma. *J Thorac Oncol* 2016; in press.
5. Rusch VW, Chansky K, Kindler HL et al. The IASLC Malignant Pleural Mesothelioma Staging Project: proposals for the M descriptors and for the revision of the TNM stage groupings in the forthcoming (eighth) edition of the TNM classification for mesothelioma. *J Thorac Oncol*, 2016; in press.

Executive Editor's Note: This chapter has been reprinted from Wittekind Ch, Compton CC, Brierley J, Sobin LH (eds) UICC TNM Supplement A Commentary on Uniform Use, fourth edition, John Wiley & Sons, Ltd., Oxford, 2012. Where needed, the text has been updated according to the 8th edition of the TNM classification of malignant pleural mesothelioma.

12

Site-Specific Explanatory Notes for Pleural Mesothelioma

There have been changes in the classification of malignant pleural mesotheliomas from the 6th edn TNM. These have been based on the analyses of the IASLC malignant pleura mesothelioma database.[1–4]

1) The staging system applies only to malignant pleural mesothelioma.
2) Regional lymph nodes include: internal mammary, intrathoracic, scalene and supraclavicular.

T1   Tumour limited to the ipsilateral parietal +/- visceral +/- mediastinal +/- diaphragmatic pleura

T2   Tumour involving each of the ipsilateral pleural surfaces (parietal, mediastinal, diaphragmatic, and visceral pleura) with at least one of the following features:
- involvement of diaphragmatic muscle
- extension of tumour from visceral pleura into the underlying pulmonary parenchyma

T3   Describes locally advanced but **potentially resectable** tumour

Tumour involving all of the ipsilateral pleural surfaces (parietal, mediastinal, diaphragmatic, and visceral pleura) with at least one of the following features:
- involvement of the endothoracic fascia
- extension into the mediastinal fat
- solitary, completely resectable focus of tumour extending into the soft tissues of the chest wall
- non-transmural involvement of the pericardium

T4	Describes locally advanced **technically unresectable** tumour
	Tumour involving all of the ipsilateral pleural surfaces (parietal, mediastinal, diaphragmatic, and visceral pleura) with at least one of the following features:
	• diffuse extension or multifocal masses of tumour in the chest wall, with or without associated rib destruction
	• direct transdiaphragmatic extension of tumour to the peritoneum
	• direct extension of tumour to the contralateral pleura
	• direct extension of tumour to mediastinal organs
	• direct extension of tumour into the spine
	• tumour extending through to the internal surface of the pericardium with or without a pericardial effusion; or tumour involving the myocardium
N1	Ipsilateral intrathoracic lymph nodes (includes ipsilateral bronchopulmonary, hilar, subcarinal, paratracheal, aortopulmonary, paraoesophageal, peridiaphragmatic, pericardial, intercostal and internal mammary nodes)
N2	Contralateral intrathoracic lymph nodes. Metastases to ipsilateral or contralateral supraclavicular lymph nodes.

References

1. Pass H, Giroux D, Kennedy C et al. The IASLC Mesothelioma database: improving staging of a rare disease through international participation. *J Thorac Oncol* 2016; in press.
2. Nowak AK, Chansky K, Rice DC et al. The IASLC Mesothelioma Staging Project: proposals for revisions of the T descriptors in the forthcoming eighth edition of the TNM classification for mesothelioma. *J Thorac Oncol* 2016; in press.
3. Rice D, Chansky K, Nowak A et al. The IASLC Mesothelioma Staging Project: proposals for revisions of the N descriptors in the forthcoming eighth edition of the TNM classification for malignant pleural mesothelioma. *J Thorac Oncol* 2016; in press.
4. Rusch VW, Chansky K, Kindler HL et al. The IASLC Malignant Pleural Mesothelioma Staging Project: proposals for the M descriptors and for the revision of the TNM stage groupings in the forthcoming (eighth) edition of the TNM classification for mesothelioma. *J Thorac Oncol*, 2016; in press.

Executive Editor's Note: This chapter has been reprinted from Wittekind Ch, Compton CC, Brierley J, Sobin LH (eds) UICC TNM Supplement A Commentary on Uniform Use, fourth edition, John Wiley & Sons, Ltd., Oxford, 2012. Where needed, the text has been updated according to the 8th edition of the TNM classification of malignant pleural mesothelioma.

13

Site-Specific Recommendations for pT and pN Categories

pT – Primary Tumour

pT3 or less
Pathological examination of the mesothelioma with *no gross tumour* at the margins of resection (with or without microscopic involvement).

pT4
Microscopic confirmation of involvement of the ipsilateral pleural surfaces, with at least one of the following:
- diffuse extension or multifocal masses of tumour in the chest wall, with or without associated rib destruction
- direct transdiaphragmatic extension of tumour to the peritoneum
- direct extension of tumour to the contralateral pleura
- direct extension of tumour to mediastinal organs
- direct extension of tumour into the spine
- tumour extending through to the internal surface of the pericardium with or without a pericardial effusion; or tumour involving the myocardium

pN – Regional Lymph Nodes

pN1
Microscopic confirmation of metastasis in ipsilateral intrathoracic lymph nodes (includes ipsilateral bronchopulmonary, hilar, subcarinal, paratracheal, aortopulmonary, paraoesophageal, peridiaphragmatic, pericardial, intercostal and internal mammary nodes).

pN2

Microscopic confirmation of metastasis in contralateral intrathoracic lymph nodes. Metastases to ipsilateral or contralateral supraclavicular lymph nodes.

Reference

1. Nowak AK, Chansky K, Rice DC et al. The IASLC Mesothelioma Staging Project: proposals for revisions of the T descriptors in the forthcoming eighth edition of the TNM classification for mesothelioma. *J Thorac Oncol* 2016; in press.
2. Rice D, Chansky K, Nowak A et al. The IASLC Mesothelioma Staging Project: proposals for revisions of the N descriptors in the forthcoming eighth edition of the TNM classification for malignant pleural mesothelioma. *J Thorac Oncol* 2016; in press.

14

Atlas of Pleural Mesothelioma Staging

T1   T2

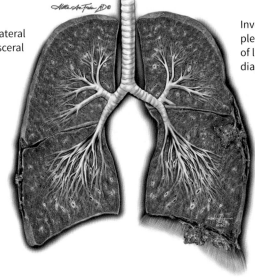

Involves ipsilateral parietal or visceral pleura only

Involves ipsilateral pleura with invasion of lung and/or diaphragmatic muscle

T3   T4

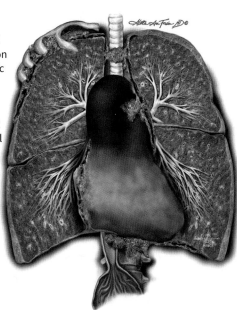

Involves ipsilateral pleura with invasion of the endothoracic fascia, the chest wall (solitary, resectable focus extending into soft tissue),mediastinal fat and/or non-transmural invasion of the pericardium

Involves ipsilateral pleura with diffuse, multifocal invasion of the chest wall, invasion of the contralateral pleura, peritoneum, mediastinal organs, spine, transmural invasion of the pericardium (with or without pericardial effusion) and/or myocardium

N1

Metastases to ipsilateral intrathoracic lymph nodes (includes ipsilateral bronchopulmonary, hilar, subcarinal, paratracheal, aortopulmonary, para-oesophageal, peridiaphragmatic, pericardial, intercostal and internal mammary lymph nodes)

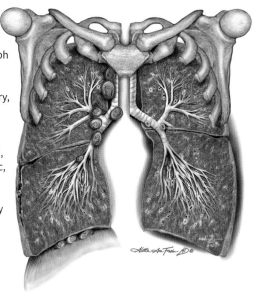

N2

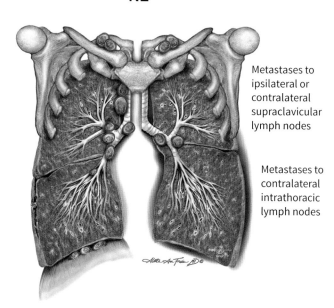

Metastases to ipsilateral or contralateral supraclavicular lymph nodes

Metastases to contralateral intrathoracic lymph nodes

PART IV

THYMIC MALIGNANCIES

15

The History of TNM Staging in Thymic Malignancies

Frank Detterbeck and Pier Luigi Filosso

History of Stage Classification of Thymic Malignancies

No official stage classification system for thymic malignancies has existed until the 8th edition of the TNM Classification of Malignant Tumours. However, at least 15 different systems have been proposed beginning in 1978, as summarized in a recent review (Table 15.1).[1] Most of these classification schemes were developed from a very limited number of patients (16-250). Most of these were never tested for prognostic discrimination in an independent dataset. These different systems achieved various levels of acceptance and use.

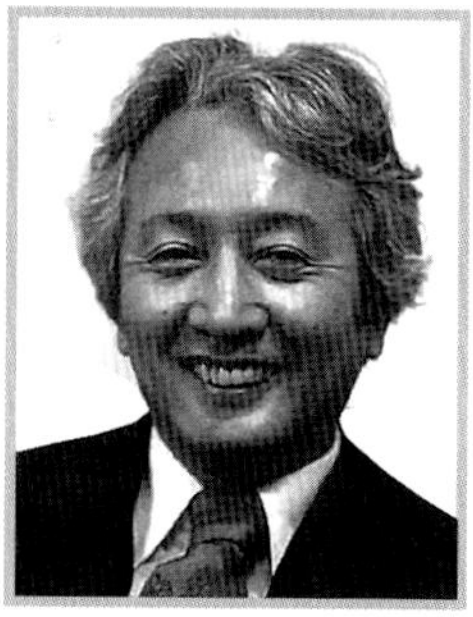

The most prominent of the stage classification systems was developed by Dr. Akira Masaoka (Figure 15.1) in 1981.[2] He was an outstanding leader in advancing the clinical science of thymic malignancies. He organized the Japanese Association for Research in the Thymus (JART), an organization that has had a huge impact on this field and continues to produce seminal contributions. The Masaoka stage classification system was based primarily on the macroscopic extent of the primary tumour. Other classification systems are often either explicit modifica-

Figure 15.1. Professor Akira Masaoka (1930-2014).

tions of the Masoaka system, or clearly used the Masaoka system as a starting point. The Masaoka system is one of the few that underwent external validation, most prominently in a national Japanese study involving 1,320 patients.[3]

Several systems included the completeness of resection in the classification, namely the Verley-Hoffmann system and that of the Groupe d'Etudes des Tumeurs Thymiques in France.[4,5] Other important aspects of particular systems are inclusion of the presence of adherence to adjacent structures[5] or tumour size and number of invaded structures.[6] Moran et al designated encapsulated tumours as stage 0.[7]

Table 15.1. Overview of previous thymic stage classification systems.

System	Year	n	Histotype	Major Feature
Non-TNM based				
Bergh[16]	1978	43	Thymoma	Capsule, invasion to other organs
Wilkins[17]	1979	103	Thymoma	Pleural/pericardial invasion in stage II
Masaoka[2]	1981	96	Thymoma	Invasion, nodes/distant metastases
Verley-Hoffmann[5]	1985	200	Thymoma	Gross invasion, R0-2
GETT[4]	1991	67	Thymoma	Gross invasion, gross degree of resection
Masoaka-Koga[18]	1994	79	Thymoma	Micro < macroscopic in stage II
ITMIG[9]	2011	—	All	Clarification of Masaoka-Koga ambiguities
Asamura[6]	2004	138	All	Size and number of invaded structures
Moran[7]	2012	250	Thymoma	Stage 0 thymoma; shifted Masaoka stages down
TNM-based				
Yamakawa[8]	1991	226	All	Defined N category; stages similar to Masaoka
Tsuchiya[19]	1994	16	TC	Stages heavily impacted by N category
WHO[20]	2004	—	All	New stage I tumors (merging "old" stages I and II)
Bedini[21]	2005	149	All	Stages driven by treatment approaches
Weissferdt[22]	2012	33	TC	Collapsed T1,2, and N groups of Yamakawa
IASLC-ITMIG[12,14]	2014	8,145	All	

GETT, Groupe d'Etudes des Tumeurs Thymiques; TC, thymic carcinoma; R0-2, completeness of resection

The Masaoka system was adapted to be a TNM-based classification by Yamakawa in 1991.[8] Other TNM based systems have generally involved modifications of this schema.[1]

The proposed systems were adopted to varying degrees by different institutions and regions. Another problem was that the systems were usually not defined in a thorough manner, leading to varying interpretations of the definitions by different institutions even when using the same classification system.[9] The inability to communicate clearly and consistently about the anatomic extent of thymic malignancies due to the lack of a uniform nomenclature was a major factor hampering progress. The need for an official stage classification system endorsed by the American Joint Committee on Cancer (AJCC) and the Union for International Cancer Control (UICC) became increasingly apparent with the emergence of collaborative efforts to foster research in thymic malignancies.

The IASLC-ITMIG Stage Classification Project
Structure of the Project

The International Thymic Malignancies Interest Group (ITMIG) and the International Association for the Study of Lung Cancer (IASLC) independently and simultaneously set out to address the need for a uniform thymic stage classification system. This soon became a joint effort, with ITMIG providing the worldwide engagement of clinicians active in this field, and IASLC providing funding and expertise from the experience of having done this in lung cancer. A Thymic Domain of the IASLC Staging and Prognostic Factors Committee (TD-SPFC) was established along with a thymic advisory board in 2010 (Table 15.2). This group represents an international multispecialty committee of recognized leaders in this field. The AJCC and UICC endorsed this initiative to develop proposals for stage classification of thymic malignancies for the 8th edition of TNM classification. The Cancer Research And Biostatistics (CRAB) organization was engaged to provide statistical expertise for the project.

The TD-SPFC established a series of guiding principles: the system would only address anatomic extent of disease, be applicable to all types of thymic malignancies, lend itself to clinical and pathologic staging and be TNM-based.[10] The process would involve analysis of worldwide data, driven primarily by recurrence of completely resected tumours in less advanced cases and overall survival regardless of resection status in more advanced cases. The group recognized that prognosis is multifactorial, influenced not only by anatomic disease extent, but also by patient factors, treatment received, patient characteristics and potentially variation by geographic region or time period. Therefore, to be considered a valid way to categorize cohorts of tumours, a classification system should have consistent discriminatory ability among subgroups and maintain significance when adjusted for other prognostic factors. Furthermore, practical considerations and similarities to lung cancer stage classification should also be taken into account, especially because the rarity of thymic malignancies poses limitations on statistical analysis.

The TD-SPFC set out to establish a database for analysis. The committee established subgroups focused on specific issues (previously proposed classification systems, T, N and M components, size, clinical staging). The findings and considerations were discussed in a series of monthly conference calls and periodic face to face meetings in 2013 and 2014. Input on emerging proposals was sought from

Table 15.2. Members of the Thymic Domain and Thymic Advisory Board of the IASLC Staging and Prognostic Factors Committee.

Name	Specialty	Institution	Location
Frank Detterbeck, chair	Thoracic surgery	Yale University	New Haven, USA
Hisao Asamura	Thoracic surgery	Keio University	Tokyo, Japan
John Crowley	Biostatistics	Cancer Research And Biostatistics	Seattle, USA
Conrad Falkson	Radiation Oncology	Queen's University	Ontario, Canada
Pier Luigi Filosso	Thoracic Surgery	University of Torino	Torino, Italy
Giuseppe Giaccone	Medical Oncology	National Cancer Institute	Bethesda, USA
Dorothy Giroux	Biostatistics	Cancer Research And Biostatistics	Seattle, USA
James Huang	Thoracic surgery	Sloan Kettering Cancer Center	New York, USA
Jhingook Kim	Thoracic surgery	Samsung Medical Center	Seoul, S Korea
Kazuya Kondo	Thoracic surgery	University of Tokushima	Tokushima, Japan
Marco Lucchi	Thoracic surgery	University of Pisa	Pisa, Italy
Mirella Marino	Pathology	Regina Elena National Cancer Institute	Rome, Italy
Edith Marom	Radiology	MD Anderson Cancer Center	Houston, USA
Alan Mitchell	Biostatistics	Cancer Research And Biostatistics	Seattle, USA
Andrew Nicholson	Pathology	Royal Brompton Hospital	London, UK
Meinoshin Okumura	Thoracic surgery	Osaka University	Osaka, Japan

the ITMIG membership as well as the entire SPFC (i.e. for all thoracic malignancies). Final proposals were published in 2014[11-14] for review by the medical community in general, and eventually accepted by the AJCC and UICC for the 8th edition manuals.

Creation of the Database

ITMIG developed an infrastructure for a global database, with development of a stage classification system targeted as one of the initial uses.[15] This was rapidly populated with 6,097 cases (after cleaning)–a testament to the culture of global collaboration that ITMIG represents. In addition, the JART contributed 2,897 cases from their database. These 8,994 cases from 77 centers in 16 countries were submitted to CRAB for analysis. An additional 1,814 cases were contributed by the European Society of Thoracic Surgeons (ESTS) thymic group directly to CRAB, resulting in a total of 10,808 cases of a thymic malignancy from 105 sites world-wide. Of these, 2663 cases were excluded (due to missing endpoints, date errors, first treatment before 1990, and other missing data), leaving 8,145 available for analysis.[14]

Most (80%) of the patients were diagnosed between 2000 and 2010, and most (76%) underwent resection (Figure 15.2). Survival status was available in all, recurrence status in 58% (4,732), and resection status in 95% (7,726) of cases. A pathologic stage was available in 99% (8,084) and clinical stage in 64% (5,232). Specific data on involved structures were available in 88% (7,197) and one dimension of size in 79% (6,441), but data on more detailed characteristics was limited.[14]

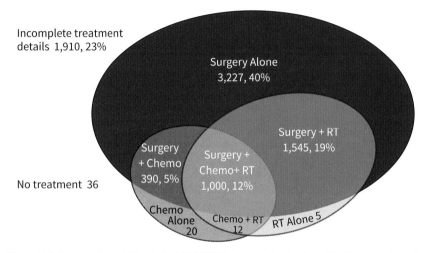

Figure 15.2. Treatment modalities in the IASLC-ITMIG retrospective database (8,145 screened cases).

Analysis and Development of Proposals for Stage Classification

The CRAB statistical group performed an extensive analysis, generating about 500 graphs, depicting outcomes by many anatomical features for various groups and subgroups. For the primary tumour, involvement of adjacent structure was grouped into several "levels" of involvement. A tumour would fall into a particular T category if one or more than one structure included in this level were involved, and whether or not structure of a lower level were involved. This provided a practical way of addressing the multitude of possible groupings stemming for the number of specific structures that could be involved either alone or in combination with others. A running log rank statistic was used to determine optimal size cutpoints, but size was not included in the final classification because it demonstrated essentially no discriminatory ability relative to various outcomes. A node map for thymic tumours was being developed by ITMIG; this was included in the work of the TD-SPFC. This map defines 2 nodal regions, an anterior perithymic region and a deep nodal region.

The discriminatory ability of candidate T, N and M categories and stage group-ings was assessed by a Cox proportional hazards regression models, adjusting for other factors. T, N and M categories and stage groups were also assessed in the entire cohort as well as specifically for thymoma only or thymic carcinoma only. After considering many possibilities and different endpoints (e.g. overall survival, recurrence, R0 patients, R-any patients) the TD-SPFC proposed the TNM system that was eventually endorsed by the UICC and AJCC and that is described in the next chapter of this manual.

Conclusion

Over several decades multiple stage classification systems had been proposed with varying degrees of adoption in different centers. Recognition of the need for an official, evidence-based classification system became increasingly apparent. An international database was created and a thymic domain of the IASLC SPFC was formed. Extensive analysis and review has led to the first official stage classification for thymic tumours adopted by the AJCC and UICC.

References

1. Filosso P, Ruffini E, Lausi P, Oliaro A, Detterbeck F. Historical perspectives: the evolution of the thymic epithelial tumors staging system. *Lung Cancer.* 2014;83(2):126-132.
2. Masaoka A, Monden Y, Nakahara K, Tanioka T. Follow-up study of thymomas with special reference to their clinical stages. *Cancer.* 1981;48:2485-2492.
3. Kondo K, Monden Y. Therapy for thymic epithelial tumors: a clinical study of 1,320 patients from Japan. *Ann Thorac Surg.* Sep 2003;76(3):878-884.
4. Gamondès JP, Balawi A, Greenland T, et al. Seventeen years of surgical treatment of thymoma: factors influencing survival. *Eur J Cardio-thorac Surg.* 1991;5:124-131.
5. Verley JM, Hollmann KH. Thymoma: A comparative study of clinical stages, histologic features, and survival in 200 cases. *Cancer.* 1985,55(5).1074-1086.
6. Asamura H, Nakagawa K, Matsuno Y, Suzuki K, Watanabe S, Tsuchiya R. Thymoma needs a new staging system. *Interac Cardiovasc and Thorac Surg.* 2004;3:163-167.
7. Moran CA, Walsh G, Suster S, Kaiser L. Thymomas II: A clinicopathologic correlation of 250 cases with a proposed staging system with emphasis on pathologic assessment. *Am J Clin Pathol.* 2012;137(3):451-461.
8. Yamakawa Y, Masaoka A, Hashimoto T, et al. A tentative tumor-node-metastasis classification of thymoma. *Cancer.* 1991;68:1984-1987.
9. Detterbeck F, Nicholson A, Kondo K, Van Schil P, Moran C. The Masaoka-Koga stage classification for thymic malignancies: clarification and definition of terms. *J Thorac Oncol.* 2011;6(7 Suppl 3):S1710-1716.
10. Detterbeck F, Asamura H, Crowley J, et al. The IASLC/ITMIG Thymic Malignancies Staging Project: development of a stage classification for thymic malignancies. *J Thorac Oncol.* 2013;8:1467-1473.
11. Bhora F, Chen D, Detterbeck F, et al. The ITMIG/IASLC Thymic Epithelial Tumors Staging Project: a proposed lymph node map for thymic epithelial tumors in the forthcoming (8th) edition of the TNM classification of malignant tumors. *J Thorac Oncol.* 2014 9 (9, supplement 2):S88-S96.
12. Detterbeck F, Stratton K, Giroux D, et al. The IASLC/ITMIG Thymic Epithelial Tumors Staging Project: proposal for an evidence-based stage classification system for the forthcoming (8th) edition of the TNM classification of malignant tumors. *J Thorac Oncol.* 2014 9 (9, Supplement 2):S65-S72.

13. Kondo K, Van Schil P, Detterbeck F, et al. The IASLC/ITMIG Thymic Epithelial Tumors Staging Project: proposals for the N and M components for the forthcoming (8th) edition of the TNM classification of malignant tumors J *Thorac Oncol.* 2014 9(9, Supplement 2):S81-S87.

14. Nicholson A, Detterbeck C, Marino M, et al. The IASLC/ITMIG Thymic Epithelial Tumors Staging Project: proposals for the T component for the forthcoming (8th) edition of the TNM classification of malignant tumors. *J Thorac Oncol.* 2014 9 (9, Supplement 2):S73-S80.

15. Huang J, Ahmad U, Antonicelli A, et al. Development of the International Thymic Malignancy Interest Group International Database: an unprecedented resource for the study of a rare tumor. *J Thorac Oncol.* 2014;9(10):1573-1578.

16. Bergh N, Gatzinsky P, Larsson S, Lundin P, Ridell B. Tumors of the thymus and thymic region; I. Clinicopathological studies on thymomas. *Ann Thorac Surg.* 1978;25:91-98.

17. Wilkins EJ, Castleman B. Thymoma: A continuing survey at the Massachusetts General Hospital. *Ann Thorac Surg.* 1979;28(3):252-256.

18. Koga K, Matsuno Y, Noguchi M, et al. A review of 79 thymomas: modification of staging system and reappraisal of conventional division into invasive and non-invasive thymoma. *Pathol Int.* 1994;44(5):359-367.

19. Tsuchiya R, Koga K, Matsuno Y, Mukai K, Shimosato Y. Thymic carcinoma: proposal for pathological TNM and staging. *Pathol Int.* 1994;44(7):505-512.

20. Travis WD, Brambilla E, Muller-Hermelink HK, Harris CC. Pathology and genetics of tumors of the lung, pleura, thymus and heart. In: Kleihues P, Sobin L, eds. *WHO Classification of Tumors.* 2nd ed: Lyon: IARC Press; 2004:145-197.

21. Bedini AV, Andreani SM, Tavecchio L, et al. Proposal of a novel system for the staging of thymic epithelial tumors. *Ann Thorac Surg.* 2005;80(6):1994-2000.

22. Weissferdt A, Moran CA. Thymic Carcinoma, Part 2: a clinicopathologic correlation of 33 cases with a proposed staging system. *Am J Clin Pathol.* 2012;138(1):115-121.

Acknowledgment: *Used with the permission of the Union for International Cancer Control (UICC), Geneva, Switzerland. The original source for this material is in Brierley JB, Gospodarowicz MK, Wittekind Ch, eds. UICC TNM Classification of Malignant Tumours, 8th edition (2017), published by John Wiley & Sons, Ltd, www.wiley.com.*

16

TNM for Thymic Malignancies

Introductory Notes

The classification applies to thymic tumours.

Each site is described under the following headings:

- Rules for classification with the procedures for assessing T, N, and M categories; additional methods may be used when they enhance the accuracy of appraisal before treatment
- Anatomical subsites where appropriate
- Definition of the regional lymph nodes
- TNM clinical classification
- pTNM pathological classification
- Stage
- Prognostic factors grid

Regional Lymph Nodes

The regional lymph nodes extend from the supraclavicular region to the diaphragm. Direct extension of the primary tumour into lymph nodes is classified as lymph node metastasis.

Thymic Tumours
ICD-0-3 C37.9

Rules for Classification

The classification applies to epithelial tumours of the thymus, including thymomas, thymic carcinomas and neuroendocrine tumours of the thymus. It does not apply to sarcomas, lymphomas and other rare tumours.

This classification is new to the 8th edition and is based upon recommendations from the International Association for the Study of Lung Cancer (IASLC) Staging Project and the International Thymic Malignancies Interest Group (ITMIG) (see references).[1-3]

There should be histological confirmation of the disease and division of cases by histological type.

The following are the procedures for assessing T, N, and M categories:

T categories   Physical examination, imaging, endoscopy, and/or surgical exploration

N categories   Physical examination, imaging, endoscopy, and/or surgical exploration

M categories   Physical examination, imaging, and/or surgical exploration

Regional Lymph Nodes

The regional lymph nodes are the anterior (perithymic) lymph nodes, the deep intrathoracic lymph nodes and the cervical lymph nodes.

TNM Clinical Classification

T – Primary Tumour

TX   Primary tumour cannot be assessed.

T0   No evidence of primary tumour

T1   Tumour encapsulated or extending into the mediastinal fat, may involve the mediastinal pleura.

    T1a   No mediastinal pleural involvement

    T1b   Direct invasion of the mediastinal pleura

T2   Tumour with direct involvement of the pericardium (partial or full thickness).

T3   Tumour with direct invasion into any of the following; lung, brachiocephalic vein, superior vena cava, phrenic nerve, chest wall, or extrapericardial pulmonary artery or vein.

T4   Tumour with direct invasion into any of the following; aorta (ascending, arch or descending), arch vessels, intrapericardial pulmonary artery, myocardium, trachea, or oesophagus

N – Regional Lymph Nodes

NX   Regional lymph nodes cannot be assessed

N0   No regional lymph node metastasis

N1   Metastasis in anterior (perithymic) lymph nodes

N2   Metastasis in deep intrathoracic or cervical lymph nodes

M – Distant Metastasis

M0   No pleural, pericardial or distant metastasis

M1   Distant metastasis
  M1a   Separate pleural or pericardial nodule(s)
  M1b   Distant metastasis beyond the pleura or pericardium

TNM Pathological Classification

The pT and pN categories correspond to the T and N categories. For pM see page 59.

Stage –Thymic Tumours

Stage I	T1	N0	M0
Stage II	T2	N0	M0
Stage IIIA	T3	N0	M0
Stage IIIB	T4	N0	M0
Stage IVA	Any T	N1	M0
	Any T	N0, N1	M1a
Stage IVB	Any T	N2	M0, M1a
	Any T	Any N	M1b

References

1. Nicholson AG, Detterbeck FC, Marino M, et al. The IASLC/ITMIG thymic epithelial tumors staging project: proposals for the T component for the forthcoming (8th) edition of the TNM classification of malignant tumors. *J Thorac Oncol* 2014; 9: s73–s80.
2. Kondo K, Van Schil P, Detterbeck FC, et al. The IASLC/ITMIG thymic epithelial tumors staging project: proposals for the N and M components for the forthcoming (8th) edition of the TNM classification of malignant tumors. *J Thorac Oncol* 2014; 9: s81–s87.
3. Detterbeck FC, Stratton K, Giroux D, et al. The IASLC/ITMIG thymic epithelial tumors staging project: proposal for an evidence-based stage classification system for the forthcoming (8th) edition of the TNM classification of malignant tumors. *J Thorac Oncol* 2014; 9: s65–s72.

17

Site-Specific Explanatory Notes for Thymic Malignancies

Frank Detterbeck

Clinical Stage Classification

1. The reliability of imaging characteristics in predicting actual invasion of mediastinal structures has generally not been defined. One must rely on the radiologist's best judgment. An elevated hemidiaphragm should be considered evidence of phrenic nerve involvement.

2. Lymph nodes ≥ 1cm in short axial dimension should be considered involved for purposes of clinical staging; similarly, nodes with PET uptake (if available) should also be considered involved.

3. A surgical exploration without microscopic confirmation of levels of invasion or the nodal status defines the clinical stage. Pathologic stage can be defined if a tumour is completely resected or if invasion of the highest T category is microscopically confirmed along with node sampling.

Pathologic Stage Classification

T Component

1. For pathologic T classification involvement of a particular tissue must be microscopically confirmed. Surgically identified adhesion of the tumour to an adjacent structure does not affect the T classification if no actual invasion of the adjacent structure is present on microscopic examination.

2. The presence or absence of a capsule or invasion thereof is not a descriptor in the T classification. The International Association for the Study of Lung Cancer-International Thymic Malignancies Interest Group (IASLC-ITMIG) analysis of a large global database demonstrated that these descriptors have no impact on outcomes.[1] This also confirms other studies.[2]

3. The impact of invasion of the mediastinal pleura is unclear. The IASLC-ITMIG database did not demonstrate a difference,[1] but a possible difference is suggested in the Japanese Association for Research on the Thymus (JART) database.[1] A problem with the analysis is that recognition of the mediastinal pleura can be difficult grossly as well as microscopically in the resected specimen. ITMIG recommends routine marking of the mediastinal pleura by the surgeon at the time of resection,[3] and the use of elastin stains is recommended when the mediastinal pleural layer is unclear microscopically.

4. Invasion of the pericardium is classified as T2 whether this is partial or full thickness.[1] The classification is the same whether there is involvement of the parietal and visceral pericardium. (There is no data suggesting a difference in outcomes, and no ability to make this distinction in clinical staging.)

5. While it is recommended that tumour size be recorded, it does not affect the T classification. In the IASLC-ITMIG global database the largest dimension of tumour size had no prognostic impact.

6. The T category is determined by the "level" of invasion. Invasion of structures of a particular T level is counted regardless whether or not there is invasion of structures of a lower level.

7. While the number of invaded mediastinal structures (of a particular level) appears to affect outcomes, this is not a factor in determining the T category. This is due to some inconsistency and a suspected variable amount of missing information regarding all of the invaded structures in the available data for analysis. It is recommended that not only is the T category recorded, but also all of the specific structures that are invaded.

8. Direct invasion of the pleura or pericardium is distinguished from pleural or pericardial nodules that are separated from the primary tumour mass (see M category notes).

N Component

1. Direct extension of the primary tumour into a lymph node is counted as nodal involvement.[4]

2. During resection of a thymoma with invasion of other structures (i.e. ≥ T2) it is recommended that anterior mediastinal nodes are routinely removed with the specimen, and systematic sampling of deep nodes in encouraged. During resection of a thymic carcinoma systematic resection of both N1 and N2 nodes is recommended. The pathologists should specifically examine and report on the presence of nodal involvement.[3-5] Furthermore, removal and specific notation of any suspicious nodes (either by imaging or intraoperative assessment) is recommended.

3. Nodal involvement is divided into an anterior (perithymic, N1) and deep (N2) category, as detailed in the ITMIG-IASLC node map (Table 17.1, 17.2 and Figures 17.1-17.6).[4,6]

Table 17.1. Anterior Region [N1] (Anterior Mediastinal & Anterior Cervical Nodes).

Region Boundaries	Node Groups[14, 16]	Node Group Boundaries
Sup: hyoid bone	Low Ant Cervical: pretracheal, paratracheal, peri-thyroid, precricoid/delphian	Sup: inferior border of cricoid
Lat (Neck): medial border of carotid sheaths		Lat: common carotid arteries
Lat (Chest): mediastinal pleura	(AAO-HNS / ASHNS level 6 / IASLC level 1)	Inf: superior border of manubrium
Ant: sternum	Peri-thymic	Proximity to thymus
Post (Medially): great vessels, pericardium	Prevascular	Sup: apex of chest
	(IASLC level 3a)	Ant: posterior sternum
Post (Laterally): phrenic nerve		Post: anterior SVC
Inf: xiphoid, diaphragm		Inf: carina
	Paraaortic, ascending aorta, superior phrenic	Sup: line tangential to sup border of aortic arch
	(IASLC level 6)	Inf: inf border of aortic arch
	Supradiaphragmatic / inferior phrenic / pericardial (along inferior poles of thymus)	Sup: inf border of aortic arch
		Ant: post sternum
		Post: phrenic nerve (laterally) or pericardium (medially)
		Inf: diaphragm

Region and node group boundaries adapted directly from definitions established by AAO-HNS, ASHNS and IASLC.

AAO-HNS, American Academy of Otolaryngology - Head and Neck Surgery; ASHNS, American Society for Head and Neck Surgery; IASLC, International Association for the Study of Lung Cancer. Sup, Superior; Ant, Anterior; Inf, inferior; Lat, lateral; Post, posterior; SVC, superior vena cava.

Table 17.2. Deep Region [N2] (Middle Mediastinal and Deep Cervical Nodes.

Region Boundaries	Node Groups[14, 16]	Node Group Boundaries
Sup: level of lower border of cricoid cartilage Anteromedial (neck): lateral border of sternohyoid, medial border of carotid sheath Posterolateral (neck): anterior border of trapezius Ant (chest): aortic arch, aortopulmonary window – anterior border of SVC Post (chest): oesophagus Lat (chest): pulmonary hila Inf: diaphragm	Lower jugular (AAO-HNS / ASHNS level 4)	Sup: level of lower border of cricoid cartilage Anteromedial: lat border of sternohyoid Posterolateral: lat border of sternocleidomastoid Inf: clavicle
	Supraclavicular/venous angle: confluence of internal jugular & subclavian vein (AAO-HNS / ASHNS level 5b)	Sup: level of lower border of cricoid cartilage Anteromedial: post border of sternocleidomastoid Posterolateral: ant border of trapezius Inf: clavicle
	Internal mammary nodes	Proximity to internal mammary arteries
	Upper paratracheal (IASLC level 2)	Sup: sup border of manubrium, apices of lungs Inf: intersection of lower border of innominate vein with trachea; sup border of aortic arch
	Lower paratracheal (IASLC level 4)	Sup: intersection of lower border of innominate vein with trachea; sup border of aortic arch Inf: lower border of azygos vein, sup border of left main pulmonary artery
	Subaortic/aortopulmonary window (IASLC level 5)	Sup: inf border of aortic arch Inf: sup border of left main pulmonary artery
	Subcarinal (IASLC level 7)	Sup: carina Inf: upper border of lower lobe bronchus on the left; lower border of the bronchus intermedius on the right
	Hilar (IASLC level 10)	Sup: lower rim of azygos vein on right, upper rim of pulmonary artery on left Inf: interlobar region bilaterally

Region and node group boundaries adapted directly from definitions established by AAO-HNS, ASHNS and IASLC.

AAO-HNS, American Academy of Otolaryngology - Head and Neck Surgery; ASHNS, American Society for Head and Neck Surgery; IASLC, International Association for the Study of Lung Cancer. Sup, Superior; Ant, Anterior; Inf, inferior; Lat, lateral; Post, posterior; SVC, superior vena cava.

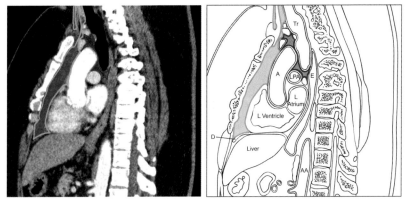

Figure 17.1. Mediastinum, Sagittal Section. Anterior region (*blue*); deep region (*purple*). Tr=trachea; E=esophagus; LPA=left pulmonary artery; A=aorta; D=diaphragm.

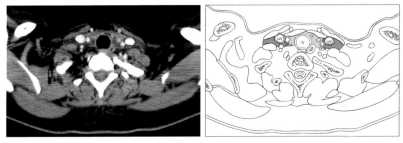

Figure 17.2. Thoracic Inlet, Axial Section. Anterior region (*blue*); deep region (*purple*). CCA=common carotid artery; IJV=internal jugular vein; Tr=trachea; Clav=clavicle; E=esophagus.

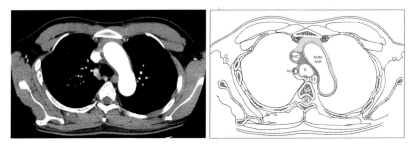

Figure 17.3. Paraaortic Level, Axial Section. Anterior region (*blue*); deep region (*purple*). SVC=superior vena cava; E=esophagus; Tr=trachea.

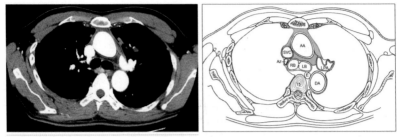

Figure 17.4. AP Window Level, Axial Section. Anterior region (*blue*); deep region (*purple*).
Note: deep region includes aortopulmonary window nodes.
AA=ascending aorta; DA=descending aorta; LPA=left pulmonary artery; SVC=superior vena
cava; Az=azygos vein; RB=right main bronchus; LB=left main bronchus.

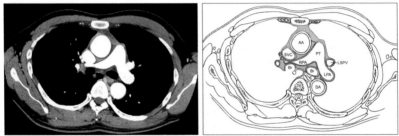

Figure 17.5. Carina Level, Axial Section. Anterior region (*blue*); deep region (*purple*).
Note: deep region includes aortopulmonary window nodes.
AA=ascending aorta; DA=descending aorta; PT=pulmonary trunk; LPA=left pulmonary artery;
RPA=right pulmonary artery; SVC=superior vena cava; LSPV=left superior pulmonary vein;
BR=bronchus; E=esophagus.

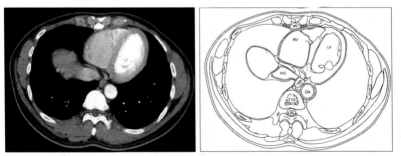

Figure 17.6. Diaphragm Level, Axial Section. Anterior region (*blue*); deep region (*purple*).
RV=right ventricle; LV=left ventricle; IVC=inferior vena cava; DA=descending aorta; E=esophagus.

M Component

1. Pleural or pericardial nodules that are separate from the primary tumor mass
   are classified as M1a.[4]
2. Discrete intraparenchymal nodules in the lung are classified as M1b. These are
   nodules of tumor that are surrounded by normal lung (i.e. not contiguous with

the visceral pleura or intraparenchymal tumor that represents direct invasion by the primary tumor mass).[4]

Resection (R) Status

The thymus is generally surrounded by loose areolar tissue, which is prone to disruption either during resection or during handling of the specimen. Furthermore, a thymectomy specimen often includes no tissues that inherently orient the specimen. Therefore, specific attention is necessary to intraoperative marking, specimen handling and orientation, and communication between the surgeon and pathologists in order to accurately report the margin status of resected tumors.[3]

1. It is suggested that immediate intraoperative marking of the specimen be performed to define areas of concern, areas of tissue disruption during handling that do not represent true margins, and specific surfaces (e.g. the right or left mediastinal pleura, areas adjacent to the innominate vein or pericardium)
2. It is recommended that the resected specimen be clearly oriented and that the margin status of specific surfaces be examined and reported (e.g. anterior, posterior, right, left, adjacent to pericardium etc.).[3] ITMIG suggests placing the specimen on a "mediastinal board" that makes the relationship of different parts of the specimen to adjacent structures clear (Figure 17.7).
3. It is recommended that the surgeon and the pathologist communicate at the time of resection about orientation and areas of particular concern
4. The distance to the nearest margin should be reported in mm whenever the margin is ≤ 3mm.

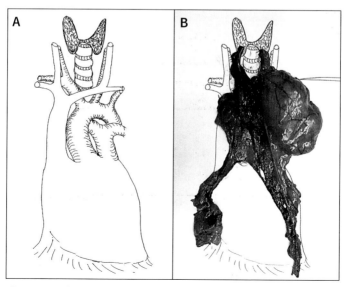

Figure 17.7. A) Mediastinal board and B) example of specimen orientation.

References

1. Nicholson A, Detterbeck C, Marino M, et al. The ITMIG/IASLC Thymic Epithelial Tumors Staging Project: proposals for the T component for the forthcoming (8th) edition of the TNM classification of malignant tumors. *J Thorac Oncol.* 2014; 9 (9, Suppl 2):S73-S80.
2. Marchevsky AM, McKenna Jr RJ, Gupta R. Thymic epithelial neoplasms: a review of current concepts using an evidence-based pathology approach. *Hematol Oncol Clin North Am.* 2008;22(3):543-562.
3. Detterbeck F, Moran C, Huang J, et al. Which way is up? Policies and procedures for surgeons and pathologicsts regarding resection specimens of thymic malignancy. *J Thorac Oncol.* 2011; 6(7 Suppl 3): S1730-S1738.
4. Kondo K, Van Schil P, Detterbeck F, et al. The IASLC/ITMIG Thymic Epithelial Tumors Staging Project: proposals for the N and M components for the forthcoming (8th) edition of the TNM classification of malignant tumors *J Thorac Oncol.* 2014; 9(9, Suppl 2):S81-S87.
5. Park IK, Kim YT, Jeon JH, et al. Importance of lymph node dissection in thymic carcinoma. *Ann Thorac Surg.* 2013; 96(3):1025-1032.
6. Bhora F, Chen D, Detterbeck F, et al. The ITMIG/IASLC Thymic Epithelial Tumors Staging Project: a proposed lymph node map for thymic epithelial tumors in the forthcoming (8th) edition of the TNM classification for malignant tumors. *J Thorac Oncol.* 2014; 9 (9, Suppl 2):S88-S96.

18

Atlas of Thymic Malignancies Staging

Axial #1

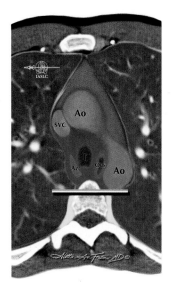

Axial #2

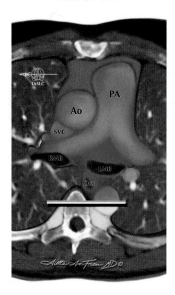

Axial #3

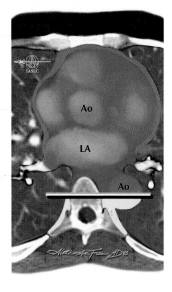

Sagittal

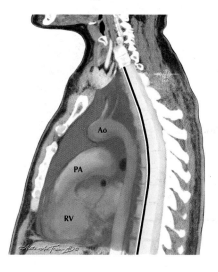

![prevascular]	Prevascular compartment	Ao: aorta
![visceral]	Visceral compartment	PA: pulmonary artery
![paravertebral]	Paravertebral compartment	SVC: superior vena cava
——	Visceral-paravertebral boundary	T: trachea

Ao: aorta
PA: pulmonary artery
SVC: superior vena cava
T: trachea
Az: azygos vein
Oes: oesophagus
RMB: right main bronchus
LMB: left main bronchus
LA: left atrium
RV: right ventricle

Stage I
T1N0M0

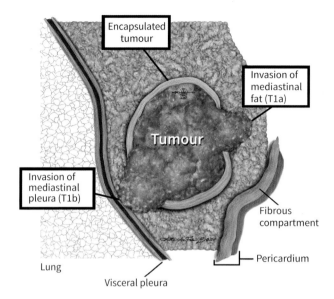

Encapsulated tumour

Invasion of mediastinal fat (T1a)

Tumour

Invasion of mediastinal pleura (T1b)

Fibrous compartment

Pericardium

Lung

Visceral pleura

Stage II
T2N0M0

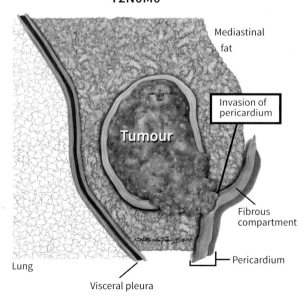

Mediastinal fat

Invasion of pericardium

Tumour

Fibrous compartment

Pericardium

Lung

Visceral pleura

Stage IIIA
T3N0M0

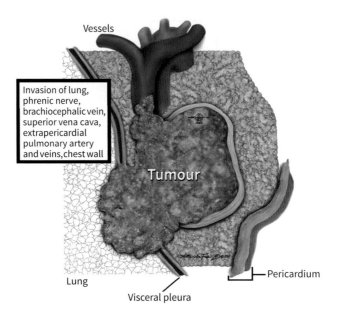

Vessels

Invasion of lung,
phrenic nerve,
brachiocephalic vein,
superior vena cava,
extrapericardial
pulmonary artery
and veins, chest wall

Tumour

Lung

Visceral pleura

Pericardium

Stage IIIB
T4N0M0

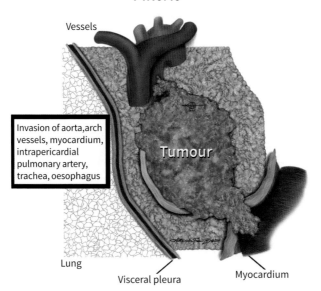

Vessels

Invasion of aorta, arch
vessels, myocardium,
intrapericardial
pulmonary artery,
trachea, oesophagus

Tumour

Lung

Visceral pleura

Myocardium

Stage IVA
Any T N1M0;
any T N0-1 M1a

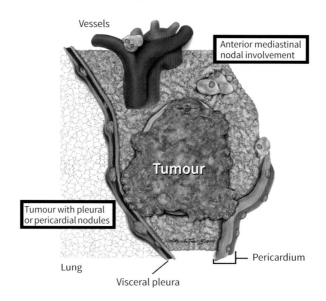

Vessels

Anterior mediastinal nodal involvement

Tumour

Tumour with pleural or pericardial nodules

Pericardium

Lung

Visceral pleura

Stage IVB
Any T N2 M0-1a;
any T, any N, M1b

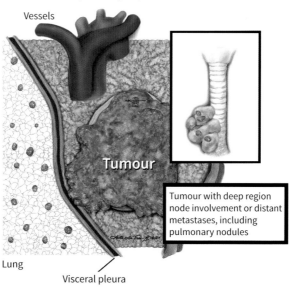

Vessels

Tumour

Tumour with deep region node involvement or distant metastases, including pulmonary nodules

Lung

Visceral pleura

PART V

CARCINOMA OF THE OESOPHAGUS AND OF OESOPHAGOGASTRIC JUNCTION

19

A Brief History of Oesophageal Cancer TNM and Stage Grouping

Thomas W. Rice and Eugene H. Blackstone

Between 1943 and 1952, Pierre Denoix of the Cancer Institute Gustave-Roussy developed the concept of TNM describing facts related to anatomic extent of a cancer. It was based on the observation that as size of an untreated primary cancer (T) increases, first regional lymph node metastases (N) and then distant metastases (M) become more frequent. In 1953, the TNM system was adopted for cancer staging. In 1958, the first recommendations for clinical staging of cancer of the breast and larynx were published.[1] It was not until 1968 that the International Union Against Cancer (UICC) published the first cancer staging manual. This was a compilation of 9 brochures that included 23 disease sites, the oesophagus being one.[2]

UICC Pocket Book 1968 and General Rules 1969

Assessment of TNM for this "1st edition of the staging manual" (1968 Pocket Book) was limited to "cases not previously treated and that the extent of the disease must be determined and recorded on clinical examination only."[2] The insistence on only clinical evaluation of all sites except for ovary (which included operative findings before definitive treatment) was stated in the complementary General Rules publication: "The condition of many patients with cancer precludes surgical treatment when they first attend for treatment. Consequently they would be excluded from a universal classification if evidence only at operation was required."[3] The differences between TNM determination and stage grouping were clearly outlined: "Classification is a means of recording facts observed by the clinician whereas staging implies interpretation of these facts regarding prognosis."[2] However, it was believed that stage grouping cancers other than breast and cervix was premature and beyond the scope of this publication. The goals of these two publications were to conduct 5-year clinical trials of the TNM systems proposed in the Pocket Book.

The first UICC oesophageal classification was proposed in 1966, with the planned 5-year trial from 1967 through 1971.[2] These staging recommendations applied only to oesophageal carcinoma. Oesophageal TNM was accessed by clinical examination, radiography, and endoscopy. The oesophagus was divided into unequal thirds, and these regions were designated as cervical, intra-thoracic, and distal, including the abdominal portion. T was defined as follows: T1, tumour confined to one region and not impairing peristalsis or motility; T2, tumour confined to one region with impaired peristalsis or motility; T3, tumour extending beyond one region; and T4, tumour extending to neighbouring structures. N was described for the cervical oesophagus only: N0, no nodes palpable; N1, movable homolateral nodes; N2, movable contralateral or bilateral nodes; and N3, fixed nodes. For intra-thoracic or abdominal regional lymph nodes, it was stated that "as it is impossible to assess the intra-thoracic and abdominal lymph nodes, the symbol NX will be used, permitting eventual addition of histological information, thus: NX- or NX+."[2] M was simply M0 if there was no clinical evidence of distant metastases and M1 if distant metastases were present.

No stage groupings were proposed for oesophageal cancer.

UICC 2nd Edition 1974

The UICC 2nd edition oesophageal recommendations were based on a review of more than 1,000 oesophageal cancer patients conducted by the American Joint Committee on Cancer (AJCC) Esophageal Task Force.[4] This work produced TNM for clinical classification, surgical evaluation classification, and post-surgical pathologic classification. UICC 2nd edition editors chose to limit TNM to clinical assessment only. Oesophageal TNM was restricted to oesophageal carcinoma with histologic confirmation. Oesophageal regions were cervical, intra-thoracic, and lower. The intra-thoracic oesophagus was further subdivided by radiographic measurements into the upper thoracic oesophagus, extending from the thoracic inlet to the lower border of the 6th thoracic vertebra (approximately 26 cm from the incisor teeth); and the mid-thoracic oesophagus, extending from the lower border of the 6th vertebra to the lower border of the 8th vertebra (approximately 31 cm from the incisor teeth). The lower oesophagus, excluded from the intra-thoracic oesophagus, extended from the lower border of the 8th thoracic vertebra to the cardia orifice (approximately 40 cm from the incisor teeth). T definitions were refined as follows: TIS, pre-invasive carcinoma; T0, no evidence of primary tumour; T1, a non-circumferential tumour of 5 cm or less in length without obstruction or extra-oesophageal invasion; T2, a tumour without extra-oesophageal spread that was either more than 5 cm in length, circumferential, or obstructing; and T3, a tumour with extra-oesophageal spread (Figure 19.1). Obstruction was confirmed either radiographically or endoscopically. Extra-oesophageal spread was determined by clinical confirmation of recurrent

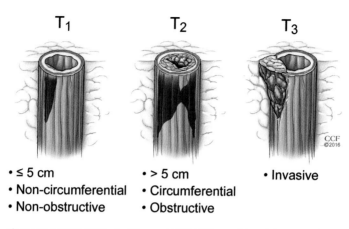

T_1 T_2 T_3

- ≤ 5 cm
- Non-circumferential
- Non-obstructive

- > 5 cm
- Circumferential
- Obstructive

- Invasive

CCF
©2016

Figure 19.1 1974 UICC 2nd edition and 1977 AJCC 1st edition definitions of T.
Copyright ©2016 Cleveland Clinic Foundation, courtesy of Thomas W. Rice, MD.

laryngeal, phrenic, or sympathetic nerve involvement, fistula formation, trachea or bronchial tree involvement, vena cava or azygos vein obstruction, or malignant effusion.

Regional lymph nodes for the cervical oesophagus were limited to cervical lymph nodes, including supraclavicular lymph nodes. For intra-thoracic oesophageal cancers, intra-abdominal and cervical lymph nodes were considered to be distant sites. Cervical regional lymph nodes were characterized as N0, no palpable nodes; N1, homolateral mobile nodes that were either not considered to contain "growth" (N1a) or considered to contain "growth" (N1b); N2, bilateral mobile nodes that were either not considered to contain "growth" (N2a) or considered to contain "growth" (N2b); and N3, fixed nodes. As in the prior publication, intra-thoracic nodes were either NX- or NX+. Distant metastases were classified as M0, no evidence of metastases, or M1, metastases to distant sites, either to distant lymph nodes (M1a) or to other sites (M1b).

Oesophageal cancer stage groupings were presented for the first time with no comment regarding how they were constructed. Stage I consisted of T1N0/N1a/N2a/NXM0, Stage II of T1N1b/N2bM0 and T2N0-2/NXM0, and Stage III of anyT3, anyN3, or anyM1.

AJCC Manual for Staging of Cancer 1977 and UICC 1978, 3rd Edition

Published in 1977, the AJCC "1st edition" Manual for Staging of Cancer introduced AJCC designated TNM definitions and, where possible, stage groupings for 18 disease sites, including the oesophagus.[5] Importantly, "general rules and the relationship between time and the staging of cancer" were introduced. These "Rules for Classification" included pre-treatment information, which was designated clinical-diagnostic staging (cTNM); information attained at surgical exploration, designated surgical-evaluation staging (sTNM); information from gross and histologic examination of the resection specimen, designated post-treatment pathologic staging (pTNM); information obtained at treatment failure and before additional treatment, designated retreatment staging (rTNM); and information found at autopsy, designated autopsy staging (aTNM).

Although not all disease sites included stage groupings, oesophageal TNM classifications were grouped and the survival basis for these stage groupings outlined in the oesophageal chapter: "The various TNM classifications can be gathered together to represent three groups of patients: 1) those patients with a fairly good prognosis when dealt with by present-day therapeutic techniques, 2) those whose course is fulminating and rapidly fatal, and 3) those whose course lies between, including those who have little or no chance of cure but who may often live for various periods."

T definitions followed those of the UICC 2nd edition (Figure 19.1). N definitions for cervical nodes were simplified from the UICC 2nd edition: N0, no palpable cervical lymph nodes; N1, palpable unilateral nodes; N2, palpable bilateral nodes; and N3, fixed nodes. N for thoracic oesophageal cancers was NX for clinical evaluation only. If surgical evaluation was used, N was simply no metastasis present (N0) or metastasis present (N1), which remained so for 32 years through six editions. Distant metastases were simply categorized as M0 (absent) or M1 (present). The sites of distant metastases were to be documented. Post-treatment residual tumour designation (R) was added to the oesophageal data form for cancer staging. R was to be recorded as R0, no residual tumour; R1, microscopic residual tumour; and R2, macroscopic residual tumour.

Non-anatomic (non-TNM) information histopathology (recorded as squamous cell carcinoma or "other" on the data form) and grade (G1, G2, G3-4), and the patient's performance status (Eastern Cooperative Oncology Group/Zubrod scale) were included in data collection recommendations.

Stage groupings were separated by primary site and reflected good (Stage I), intermediate (Stage II), and poor survival (Stage III). Stage groupings for the cervical oesophagus were Stage I, which consisted of "TIS"-1N0M0; Stage II, T1N1-2M0 and T2N0-2M0; and Stage III, anyT3, anyN3, and anyM1. For the thoracic oesophagus, Stage I was TIS-1N0-XM0; Stage II, T2N0-XM0; and Stage III, anyT3, anyN1, and anyM1 (Figure 19.2).

The UICC 3rd edition required histologic confirmation of the cancer, and any unconfirmed cases were to be reported separately.[6] Information derived from surgical exploration before definitive treatment was deemed clinical information, but this additional source of information was to be recorded. TIS was changed to Tis. cTNM definitions were identical to those in the AJCC 1st edition. Post-surgical pTNM was added to the manual. Importantly, pT was defined for the first time by depth of

	TIS	T1	T2	T3
N0	I	I	II	III
N1	III	III	III	III
M1	III	III	III	III

Figure 19.2. 1977 AJCC 1st edition stage groupings for thoracic oesophageal cancer.

primary tumour invasion: pTis, pre-invasive carcinoma (carcinoma in situ); pT1, invasion limited to the mucosa or submucosa; pT2, invasion limited to the muscle coat; and pT3, invasion beyond the muscle coat (pT3a) or into adjacent structures (pT3b). pN mirrored cN for cervical cancers, but was defined as pN0 (no regional lymph node metastasis) and pN1 (regional lymph node metastasis) for the intra-thoracic oesophagus if surgical evaluation was performed.

Stage groupings for the cervical oesophagus and intra-thoracic oesophagus were similar to those of the AJCC 1st edition, except that Stage IV was added and restricted to M1 cancers.

UICC 3rd Edition Enlarged and Revised 1982 and AJCC 2nd Edition 1983

The UICC revised and enlarged 3rd edition oesophageal recommendations were unchanged from the original 3rd edition.[7] The 2nd edition AJCC cancer staging manual was published in 1983 and added post-surgical primary tumour (pT) and distant metastasis (pM) definitions similar to those in the UICC 3rd editions. pN definitions were unique to this publication: pN0, regional nodes not involved; pN1, unilateral regional nodes involved; pN2, bilateral regional nodes involved; and pN3, extensive multiple regional nodes involved.

In the AJCC manual, Stage 0 (cTis) and Stage IV (cM1 and pM1) were added.[8] In addition, 5-year survival was presented for the stage group I-IV; excellent 83%, fair 46%, poor 26%, and distant spread 7%.[9]

UICC 1987 Fully Revised 4th Edition and AJCC 1988 3rd Edition

The 1987 UICC fully revised 4th edition[10] and 1988 AJCC 3rd edition[11] staging manuals further refined oesophageal cancer staging. Anatomic subsites were revised for the intra-thoracic oesophagus. The upper thoracic oesophagus was described as extending from the thoracic inlet to the tracheal bifurcation, the distal margin being approximately 24 cm from the upper incisor teeth. The middle thoracic oesophagus was defined as the proximal half of the oesophagus extending from the tracheal bifurcation to the oesophagogastric junction, the distal margin being approximately 32 cm from the upper incisor teeth. The lower thoracic oesophagus was defined as the distal half of the oesophagus extending from the tracheal bifurcation to the oesophagogastric junction, the distal margin being approximately 40 cm from the upper incisor teeth. T changes included substituting the term muscularis propria for muscle coat for T2 cancers, restricting T3 to cancers invading the oesophageal adventitia, and adding T4 cancers invading adjacent structures (Figure 19.3). Regional lymph nodes for the thoracic oesophagus now included perigastric nodes but not celiac nodes. N was simplified for all regions: N0, no regional lymph node metastasis; N1, regional lymph node metastasis; and NX, regional lymph nodes cannot be assessed.

Histologic grade G3-4 was separated and reported as G3 (poorly differentiated) and G4 (undifferentiated).

Stage groupings were revised and expanded by adding Stage II subgroups. Stage 0 consisted of TisN0M0; Stage I, T1N0M0; Stage IIA, pT2-3N0M0; Stage IIB, pT1-2N1M0; Stage III, T3N1M0 and T4anyNM0; and Stage IV, any M1 (Figure 19.4).

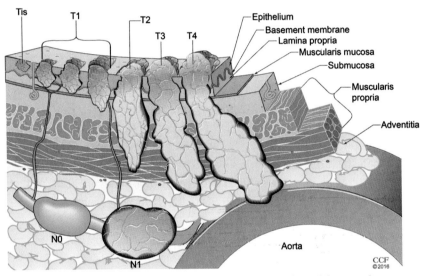

Figure 19.3. 1987 UICC fully revised 4th edition and 1988 AJCC 3rd edition definitions of T and N. Copyright ©2016 Cleveland Clinic Foundation, courtesy of Thomas W. Rice, MD.

UICC 1992 4th Edition Second Revision and AJCC 1992 4th Edition

There were no changes in oesophageal cancer staging in the 1992 4th editions.[12,13] However, the AJCC manual included a survival curve of 5,071 Japanese oesophageal

	T1	T2	T3	T4
N0	I	IIA	IIA	III
N1	IIB	IIB	III	III
M1	IV	IV	IV	IV

Figure 19.4. 1987 UICC fully revised 4th edition and 1988 AJCC 3rd edition stage groupings.

cancer patients according to 4th edition stage groupings for oesophageal cancer.[14]

UICC and AJCC 1997 5th Editions

A milestone was reached in 1997 when, after 7 UICC and 4 AJCC publications, the 5th editions were published simultaneously.[15,16] The 5th editions introduced the subclassification of M1 into M1a (cervical lymph node metastases for cancers of the upper thoracic oesophagus and celiac lymph node metastasis for cancer of the lower thoracic oesophagus) and M1b (all other distant site metastases).

The AJCC manual listed prognostic factors, including location in the lower thoracic oesophagus and adenocarcinoma histologic cell type for pT1 cancers, which were associated with better survival compared to upper and middle thoracic oesophageal location and squamous cell carcinoma cell type.

Stage IV subgroups Stage IVA (M1a) and Stage IVB (M1b) were necessary because of the addition of M subclassification. In the AJCC manual, the basic rules for stage grouping were given: Survival must be distinctive between stage groups and homogeneous within groups.

UICC and AJCC 2002 6th Editions

The 6th editions of 2002 were essentially unchanged from the 5th editions.[17,18] The AJCC manual included a regional lymph node map with numbering of specific lymph node stations.

UICC and AJCC 2009 7th Editions

At the request of the AJCC, the Worldwide Esophageal Cancer Collaboration (WECC) was inaugurated in 2006. Data collected from 13 institutions in five countries and three continents were used to construct a database of 4,627 oesophagectomy patients who had not received induction or adjuvant therapy.[19] These data served as the substrate for a modern machine learning Random Forest analysis that produced stage groupings with monotonically decreasing risk-adjusted survival with increasing stage group, distinctive risk-adjusted survival between groups, and homogeneous risk-adjusted survival within groups.[20,21] These served as the bases for the UICC and AJCC 7th edition staging manuals.[22,23]

Seventh edition TNM definitions are listed in Table 19.1. The criteria for Tis and T4 cancers were revised. Tis was redefined as high-grade dysplasia and included all non-invasive neoplastic epithelium that was previously called carcinoma *in situ*. T4 cancers were subcategorized as T4a and T4b; T4a was a resectable cancer invading adjacent structures such as pleura, pericardium, or diaphragm, and T4b was an unresectable cancer invading other adjacent structures, such as aorta, vertebral body, and trachea. A regional lymph node was redefined to include any para-oesophageal node extending from peri-oesophageal cervical nodes to celiac nodes. N was based on number of cancer-positive nodes: N0, no cancer-positive nodes; N1, 1–2 cancer-positive nodes; N2, 3–6 cancer-positive nodes; and N3, 7 or more cancer-positive nodes. The subcategories M1a and M1b were eliminated, as was MX. Metastases to distant sites were simply designated M0, no distant metastasis; and M1, distant metastasis.

In the 7th edition, non-anatomic categories histopathologic cell type, histologic grade, and tumour location were identified as important for early stage grouping (Table 19.1). Increasing histologic grade was associated with incrementally decreasing survival for T1N0M0 carcinomas, while increasing grade and upper and middle thoracic oesophageal location were associated with worse survival for T2-3N0M0 squamous cell carcinomas.

The 7th edition harmonized staging of cancer across the oesophagogastric junction. Previous staging produced different stage groupings for these cancers, depending on use of either oesophageal or gastric stage groupings. Seventh edition staging was for cancers of the oesophagus and eosophagogastric junction and included cancer within the first 5 cm of the stomach (cardia) that invade the oesophagogastric junction (Siewert III).

Seventh edition stage groupings are illustrated in Figures 19.5 and 19.6. Stages 0 and IV were by definition (not data driven) TisN0M0 and T any N any M1, respectively. The difference in survival between adenocarcinoma and squamous cell carcinoma was best managed by separate stage groupings for stages I and II. For T1N0M0 and T2N0M0, adenocarcinoma subgrouping was by histologic grade: G1 and G2 (not G3) versus G3. For T1N0M0 squamous cell carcinoma, subgrouping was by histologic grade: G1 versus G2-3. For T2N0M0 and T3N0M0 squamous cell carcinoma, stage grouping was by histologic grade and location. The four combinations ranged from G1 lower thoracic squamous cell carcinoma (Stage IB), which had the best survival, to G2-G3 upper and middle thoracic squamous cell carcinomas (Stage IIB), which had the worst. G2-G3 lower thoracic squamous cell carcinomas and G1 upper and middle thoracic squamous cell carcinomas were grouped together (Stage IIA), with intermediate survival. Stages 0, III, and IV adenocarcinoma and squamous cell carcinoma were identically stage grouped. Adenosquamous carcinomas were staged as squamous cell carcinomas, and G4 (undifferentiated) carcinomas were staged as G3 squamous cell carcinomas.

Preparation for 8th Editions

From 33 WECC institutions in 6 continents and 13 countries, data for 22,654 patients with epithelial oesophageal cancers were obtained. This effort collected 39 variables for future risk adjustment. A total of 22,123 patients had clinical staging before treatment decision,[24] 13,300 had pathologic staging after oesophagectomy or endoscopic treatment without preoperative therapy,[25] and 7,773 had pathologic staging after neoadjuvant therapy.[26] These data served as the substrate for the machine

Table 19.1: 2009 UICC and AJCC 7th Edition TNM and Non-anatomic Definitions.

Primary Tumour (T)

TX   Primary tumour cannot be assessed

T0   No evidence of primary tumour

Tis   High-grade dysplasia[†]

T1   Tumour invades lamina propria, muscularis mucosae, or submucosa

      T1a   Tumour invades lamina propria or muscularis mucosae

      T1b   Tumour invades submucosa

T2   Tumour invades muscularis propria

T3   Tumour invades adventitia

T4   Tumour invades adjacent structures

      T4a   Resectable tumour invading pleura, pericardium, or diaphragm

      T4b   Unresectable tumour invading other adjacent structures, such as aorta, vertebral body, trachea, etc.

Regional Lymph Nodes (N)[‡]

NX   Regional lymph nodes cannot be assessed

N0   No regional lymph node metastasis

N1   Regional lymph node metastases involving 1 to 2 nodes

N2   Regional lymph node metastases involving 3 to 6 nodes

N3   Regional lymph node metastases involving 7 or more nodes

Distant Metastasis (M)

MX   Distant metastasis cannot be assessed

M0   No distant metastasis

M1   Distant metastasis

Histopathologic Type

Squamous cell carcinoma

Adenocarcinoma

Histologic Grade (G)

GX   Grade cannot be assessed—stage grouping as G1

G1   Well differentiated

G2   Moderately differentiated

G3   Poorly differentiated

G4   Undifferentiated—stage grouping as G3 squamous

continued on next page

Location§

Upper or middle—cancers above lower border of inferior pulmonary vein

Lower—below inferior pulmonary vein

†Includes all non-invasive neoplastic epithelium that was previously called carcinoma in situ. Cancers stated to be non-invasive or in situ are classified as Tis.

‡Number must be recorded for total number of regional nodes sampled and total number of reported nodes with metastases.

§Location (primary cancer site) is defined by position of upper (proximal) edge of tumour in oesophagus.

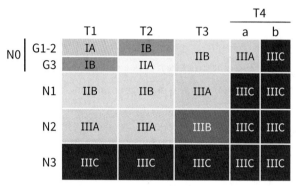

Figure 19.5. 2009 UICC and AJCC 7th edition stage groupings for adenocarcinoma of the oesophagus.

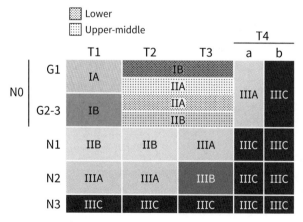

Figure 19.6. 2009 UICC and AJCC 7th edition stage groupings for squamous cell carcinoma of the oesophagus.

learning analysis that produced recommendations for oesophageal cancer stage grouping in the upcoming 8th edition cancer staging manuals.

A Perspective

TNM was proposed as a method of describing the anatomic extent of a cancer at presentation. Early on it was realized that "interpretation of these facts regarding prognosis" permitted stage grouping. Further evolution of staging theory allowed this two-step process to be applied at various times during treatment of a cancer. The cycle of review and revision has permitted modification of TNM categories and, for certain cancers, cautious introduction of non-anatomic categories.

As a description of the anatomic extent of a cancer, TNM continues to have great relevance in cancer patient care. The role of stage groupings derived from prognosis based on TNM and limited non-anatomic cancer characteristics has less relevance for the individual patient, particularly as the age of precision cancer care is upon us. However, stage grouping remains important for communication, research, and coarse prognostication for patient groups.

References

1. International Union Against Cancer (UICC). Committee on Clinical Stage Classification and Applied Statistics of Malignant Tumors. Clinical Stage Classification and Presentation of Results, Malignant Tumors of the Breast and Larynx. Paris; 1958.
2. International Union Against Cancer (UICC). TNM Classification of Malignant Tumors. Geneva; 1968.
3. International Union Against Cancer (UICC). TNM General Rules. Geneva; 1969.
4. International Union Against Cancer (UICC). TNM Classification of Malignant Tumors, 2nd edition. Geneva; 1974.
5. Manual for Staging of Cancer 1977. American Joint Committee for Cancer Staging and End-Results Reporting. Chicago; 1977.
6. International Union Against Cancer (UICC). TNM Classification of Malignant Tumors, 3rd edition. Harmer MH, ed. Geneva; 1978.
7. Harmer MH, ed. International Union Against Cancer (UICC). TNM Classification of Malignant Tumors, 3rd Edition Enlarged and Revised 1982. Geneva; 1982.
8. Beahrs OH, Meyers MH, eds. Manual for Staging of Cancer, 2nd edition. Philadelphia: J.B. Lippincott; 1983.
9. Huang GJ, Zhang DW, Wang GQ, et al. Surgical treatment of carcinoma of the esophagus: report of 1,647. *Chin Med J* (Engl). 1981;94:305-7.
10. Hermanek P, Sobin LH, eds. International Union Against Cancer (UICC). TNM Classification of Malignant Tumors, 4th Fully Revised Edition. Berlin: Springer-Verlag; 1987.
11. Beahrs OH, Henson DE, Hutter RVP, Meyers MH, eds. Manual for Staging of Cancer, 3rd edition. Philadelphia: J.B. Lippincott; 1987.
12. Hermanek P, Sobin LH, eds. International Union Against Cancer (UICC). TNM Classification of Malignant Tumors, 4th edition, 2nd revision. Berlin: Springer-Verlag; 1992.
13. Beahrs OH, Henson DE, Hutter RVP, Kennedy BJ, eds. Manual for Staging of Cancer, 4th edition. Philadelphia: J.B. Lippincott; 1992.
14. Iizuka T, Isono K, Kakegawa T, Watanabe H. Parameters linked to ten-year survival in Japan of resected esophageal carcinoma. Japanese Committee for Registration of Esophageal Carcinoma Cases. *Chest*. 1989;96:1005-11.

15. Sobin LH, Wittekind C, eds. International Union Against Cancer (UICC). TNM Classification of Malignant Tumors, 5th edition. New York: John Wiley & Sons; 1997.

16. Fleming ID, Cooper JS, Henson DE, et al., eds. AJCC Cancer Staging Manual, 5th edition. Philadelphia: Lippincott-Raven; 1997.

17. Sobin LH, Wittekind C, eds. International Union Against Cancer (UICC). TNM Classification of Malignant Tumors, 6th edition. New York: Wiley-Liss; 2002.

18. Greene FL, Page DL, Fleming ID, et al., eds. AJCC Cancer Staging Manual, 6th edition. New York: Springer-Verlag; 2002.

19. Rice TW, Rusch VW, Apperson-Hansen C, et al. Worldwide Esophageal Cancer Collaboration. *Dis Esophagus*. 2009;22:1-8.

20. Ishwaran H, Blackstone EH, Apperson-Hansen C, Rice TW. A novel approach to cancer staging: application to esophageal cancer. *Biostatistics* 2009;10:603-20.

21. Rice TW, Rusch VW, Ishwaran H, Blackstone EH. Cancer of the esophagus and esophagogastric junction: data-driven staging for the 7th edition of the American Joint Committee on Cancer/ International Union Against Cancer Staging Manuals. *Cancer*. 2010;116:3763-73.

22. Sobin LH, Gospodarowicz MK, Wittekind C, eds. International Union Against Cancer (UICC). TNM Classification of Malignant Tumors, 7th edition. New York: Wiley-Blackwell; 2009.

23. Edge SB, Byrd DR, Compton CC, Fritz AG, Greene FL, Trotti A 3rd, eds. AJCC Cancer Staging Manual, 7th edition. New York: Springer-Verlag; 2009.

24. Rice TW, Apperson-Hansen C, DiPaola LM, et al. Worldwide Esophageal Cancer Collaboration: clinical staging data. *Dis Esophagus*. 2016;7:707-14.

25. Rice TW, Chen L-Q, Hofstetter WL, et al. Worldwide Esophageal Cancer Collaboration: pathologic staging data. *Dis Esophagus*. 2016;7:724-33.

26. Rice TW, Lerut TEMR, Orringer MB, et al. Worldwide Esophageal Cancer Collaboration: neoadjuvant pathologic staging data. *Dis Esophagus*. 2016;7:715-23.

Acknowledgment: Used with the permission of the Union for International Cancer Control (UICC), Geneva, Switzerland. The original source for this material is in Brierley JB, Gospodarowicz MK, Wittekind Ch, eds. UICC TNM Classification of Malignant Tumours, 8th edition (2017), published by John Wiley & Sons, Ltd, www.wiley.com. There are some differences between the published 8th editions of the TNM classification of carcinoma of the oesophagus and of the oesophagogastric junction published by the UICC and the American Joint Committee on Cancer. The Editorial Addendum following this chapter explains these differences.

20

8th Edition of TNM for Carcinoma of the Oesophagus and of the Oesophagogastric Junction

Rules for Classification

The classification applies only to carcinomas and includes adenocarcinomas of the oesophagogastric/gastroesophageal junction. There should be histological confirmation of the disease and division of cases by topographic localization and histological type. A tumour the epicentre of which is within 2 cm of the **oesophagogastric junction** and also extends into the oesophagus is classified and staged using the oesophageal scheme. Cancers involving the oesophagogastric junction (OGJ) whose epicentre is within the proximal 2 cm of the cardia (Siewert types I/II) are to be staged as oesophageal cancers.

The following are the procedures for assessing T, N, and M categories:

T categories   Physical examination, imaging, endoscopy, (including bronchoscopy), and/or surgical exploration

N categories   Physical examination, imaging, and/or surgical exploration

M categories   Physical examination, imaging, and/or surgical exploration

Anatomical Subsites

1. Cervical oesophagus (C15.0): this commences at the lower border of the cricoid cartilage and ends at the thoracic inlet (suprasternal notch), approximately 18 cm from the upper incisor teeth.
2. Intrathoracic oesophagus
   a) The upper thoracic portion (C15.3) extending from the thoracic inlet to the level of the tracheal bifurcation, approximately 24 cm from the upper incisor teeth.
   b) The mid-thoracic portion (C15.4) is the proximal half of the oesophagus between the tracheal bifurcation and the oesophagogastric junction. The lower level is approximately 32 cm from the upper incisor teeth.

c) The lower thoracic portion (C15.5), approximately 8 cm in length (includes abdominal oesophagus), is the distal half of the oesophagus between the tracheal bifurcation and the oesophagogastric junction. The lower level is approximately 40 cm from the upper incisor teeth.

3. Oesophagogastric junction (C16.0). Cancers involving the oesophagogastric junction (OGJ) whose epicentre is within the proximal 2 cm of the cardia (Slewert types I/II) are to be staged as oesophageal cancers. Cancers whose epicentre is more than 2 cm distal from the OGJ will be staged using the Stomach Cancer TNM and Stage even if the OGJ is involved.

Regional Lymph Nodes

The regional lymph nodes, irrespective of the site of the primary tumour, are those in the oesophageal drainage area including coeliac axis nodes and paraesophageal nodes in the neck but not the supraclavicular nodes.

TNM Clinical Classification

T – Primary Tumour

TX   Primary tumour cannot be assessed
T0   No evidence of primary tumour
Tis   Carcinoma *in situ*/high-grade dysplasia
T1   Tumour invades lamina propria, muscularis mucosae, or submucosa
      T1a   Tumour invades lamina propria or muscularis mucosae
      T1b   Tumour invades submucosa
T2   Tumour invades muscularis propria
T3   Tumour invades adventitia
T4   Tumour invades adjacent structures
      T4a.   Tumour invades pleura, pericardium, azygos vein, diaphragm, or peritoneum
      T4b.   Tumour invades other adjacent structures such as aorta, vertebral body, or trachea

N – Regional Lymph Nodes

NX   Regional lymph nodes cannot be assessed
N0   No regional lymph node metastasis
N1   Metastasis in 1 to 2 regional lymph nodes
N2   Metastasis in 3 to 6 regional lymph nodes
N3   Metastasis in 7 or more regional lymph nodes

M – Distant Metastasis

M0   No distant metastasis
M1   Distant metastasis

pTNM Pathological Classification

The pT and pN categories correspond to the T and N categories. For pM see page 59.

pN0 Histological examination of a regional lymphadenectomy specimen will ordinarily include 7 or more lymph nodes. If the lymph nodes are negative, but the number ordinarily examined is not met, classify as pN0.

Stage and Prognostic Group – Carcinomas of the Oesophagus and Oesophagogastric Junction*

Squamous Cell Carcinoma

Clinical Stage

Stage 0	Tis	N0	M0
Stage I	T1	N0, N1	M0
Stage II	T2	N0, N1	M0
	T3	N0	M0
Stage III	T1, T2	N2	M0
	T3	N1, N2	M0
Stage IVA	T4a, T4b	N0, N1, N2	M0
	Any T	N3	M0
Stage IVB	Any T	Any N	M1

Pathological Stage

Stage 0	Tis	N0	M0
Stage IA	T1a	N0	M0
Stage IB	T1b	N0	M0
Stage IIA	T2	N0	M0
Stage IIB	T1	N1	M0
	T3	N0	M0
Stage IIIA	T1	N2	M0
	T2	N1	M0
Stage IIIB	T2	N2	M0
	T3	N1, N2	M0
	T4a	N0, N1	M0
Stage IVA	T4a	N2	M0
	T4b	Any N	M0
	Any T	N3	M0
Stage IVB	Any T	Any N	M1

Pathological Prognostic Group

Group	T	N	M	Grade	Location
Group 0	Tis	N0	M0	N/A	Any
Group IA	T1a	N0	M0	1, X	Any
Group IB	T1a	N0	M0	2–3	Any
	T1b	N0	M0	Any	Any
	T2	N0	M0	1	Any
Group IIA	T2	N0	M0	2–3, X	Any
	T3	N0	M0	Any	Lower
	T3	N0	M0	1	Upper, middle
Group IIB	T3	N0	M0	2–3	Upper, middle
	T3	N0	M0	Any	X
	T3	N0	M0	X	Any
	T1	N1	M0	Any	Any
Group IIIA	T1	N2	M0	Any	Any
	T2	N1	M0	Any	Any
Group IIIB	T2	N2	M0	Any	Any
	T3	N1, N2	M0	Any	Any
	T4a	N0, N1	M0	Any	Any
Group IVA	T4a	N2	M0	Any	Any
	T4b	Any N	M0	Any	Any
	Any T	N3	M0	Any	Any
Group IVB	Any T	Any N	M1	Any	Any

Adenocarcinoma

Clinical Stage

Stage 0	Tis	N0	M0
Stage I	T1	N0	M0
Stage IIA	T1	N1	M0
Stage IIB	T2	N0	M0
Stage III	T2	N1	M0
	T3, T4a	N0, N1	M0
Stage IVA	T1–T4a	N2	M0
	T4b	N0, N1, N2	M0
	Any T	N3	M0
Stage IVB	Any T	Any N	M1

Pathological Stage

Stage	T	N	M
Stage 0	Tis	N0	M0
Stage IA	T1a	N0	M0
Stage IB	T1b	N0	M0
Stage IIA	T2	N0	M0
Stage IIB	T1	N1	M0
	T3	N0	M0
Stage IIIA	T1	N2	M0
	T2	N1	M0
Stage IIIB	T2	N2	M0
	T3	N1, N2	M0
	T4a	N0, N1	M0
Stage IVA	T4a	N2	M0
	T4b	Any N	M0
	Any T	N3	M0
Stage IVB	Any T	Any N	M1

Pathological Prognostic Group

Group	T	N	M	Grade
Group 0	Tis	N0	M0	N/A
Group IA	T1a	N0	M0	1, X
Group IB	T1a	N0	M0	2
	T1b	N0	M0	1, 2, X
Group IC	T1a, T1b	N0	M0	3
	T2	N0	M0	1, 2
Group IIA	T2	N0	M0	3, X
Group IIB	T1	N1	M0	Any
	T3	N0	M0	Any
Group IIIA	T1	N2	M0	Any
	T2	N1	M0	Any
Group IIIB	T2	N2	M0	Any
	T3	N1, N2	M0	Any
	T4a	N0, N1	M0	Any
Group IVA	T4a	N2	M0	Any
	T4b	Any N	M0	Any
	Any T	N3	M0	Any
Group IVB	Any T	Any N	M1	Any

Note
*The AJCC publishes prognostic groups for adenocarcinoma and squamous cell carcinoma after neoadjuvant therapy (categories with the prefix "y"). See the Executive Editor's Note at the end of this chapter.

Prognostic Factors Grid – Oesophagus

Prognostic factors for survival in oesophageal cancer

Prognostic Factors	Tumour Related	Host Related	Environment Related
Essential	Depth of invasion Lymph node involvement Presence of lymphovascular invasion (LVI)	Performance status Age Nutritional status	Quality of surgery Multimodality approach
Additional	Tumour grading Tumour location	Economic status	Nutritional support
New and promising	CEA, VEGF-C, HER 2		

Source: *UICC Manual of Clinical Oncology*, Ninth Edition. Edited by Brian O'Sullivan, James D. Brierley, Anil K. D'Cruz, Martin F. Fey, Raphael Pollock, Jan B. Vermorken and Shao Hui Huang. © 2015 UICC. Published 2015 by John Wiley & Sons, Ltd.

Editorial Addendum

By Thomas W. Rice, MD, and Eugene H. Blackstone, MD

The 8th editions of the cancer staging manuals for carcinoma of the oesophagus and of the oesophagogastric junction[1,2] are based on modern machine learning analyses of 22,654 patients registered by the Worldwide Esophageal Cancer Collaboration (WECC).[3-8] The Union for International Cancer Control (UICC) definitions vary somewhat from those used to develop the staging recommendations and some categories are undefined by the UICC.

Location (Anatomic Subsites)

The definitions of anatomic subsites (location) used by the UICC differ from that used by the American Joint Committee on Cancer (AJCC) and WECC to develop the staging recommendations. The boundaries used to define the cervical, upper thoracic, middle thoracic and lower thoracic esophagus are defined in Table 1. The AJCC Upper GI Task Force consensus redefined the oesophagogastric junction, such that tumours with epicentres no more than 2 cm into the proximal stomach are staged as oesophageal cancers.

Table 1. Anatomic subsites (location category), defined by the position of the epicentre of the tumour in the oesophagus[1]

Location Category	Definition
X	Location unknown
Cervical	Inferior border of the hypopharynx to sternal notch, 15 cm to 20 cm[#]
Upper	Sternal notch to lower border of azygos vein, >20 cm to 25 cm[#]
Middle	Lower border of azygos vein to lower border of inferior pulmonary veins, >25 cm to 30 cm[#]
Lower	Lower border of inferior pulmonary vein to stomach, including gastroesophageal junction, >30 cm to 40 cm[#]

\# Typical measurements from the incisor teeth.

Histologic Grade

Crucial to pathological staging of early squamous cell carcinoma and adenocarcinoma of the oesophagus is the non-anatomic cancer category histologic grade. The definitions suggested for use with these staging recommendations are listed in Tables 2 and 3.

Stage Groups

Analyses of WECC data[6-8] demonstrated the need for separate stage groupings based on AJCC defined classifications (clinical, pathological, and postneoadju-

Table 2. Histologic grade (G category) for squamous cell carcinoma[*]

G Category	Criteria
G1	Well-differentiated. Prominent keratinization with pearl formation and a minor component of nonkeratinizing basal-like cells. Tumour cells are arranged in sheets, and mitotic counts are low.
G2	Moderately differentiated. Variable histologic features, ranging from para-keratotic to poorly keratinizing lesions. Generally, pearl formation is absent.
G3	Poorly differentiated. Consists predominantly of basal-like cells forming large and small nests with frequent central necrosis. The nests consist of sheets or pavement-like arrangements of tumour cells, and occasionally are punctuated by small numbers of parakeratotic or keratinizing cells. If further testing of "undifferentiated" cancers reveals a squamous cell component, or if after further testing they remain undifferentiated, categorize as squamous cell carcinoma, G3.

[*]Reproduced with permission and adapted from Rice TW, Ishwaran H, Ferguson MK, Blackstone EH, Goldstraw P. Cancer of the esophagus and esophagogastric junction: an 8th edition staging primer. *J Thorac Oncol* 2016; in press.[9]

Table 3. Histologic grade (G category) for adenocarcinoma[*]

G Category	Criteria
G1	Well differentiated. >95% of tumour is composed of well-formed glands.
G2	Moderately differentiated. 50% to 95% of tumour shows gland formation.
G3	Poorly differentiated. Tumours composed of nest and sheets of cells with <50% of tumour demonstrating glandular formation. If further testing of "undifferentiated" cancers reveals a glandular component, categorize as adenocarcinoma G3.

[*]Reproduced with permission and adapted from Rice TW, Ishwaran H, Ferguson MK, Blackstone EH, Goldstraw P. Cancer of the esophagus and esophagogastric junction: an 8th edition staging primer. *J Thorac Oncol* 2016; in press.[9]

vant therapy).[1] Additionally separate groupings for histopathologic cell type were required for clinically staged and pathologically staged tumours. UICC adopted *Clinical Stage Groups* in an unaltered state. The UICC listing of *Pathologic Stage Groups* for squamous cell carcinoma and adenocarcinoma without histologic grade and location, which are identical for both histopathologic cell types in this analysis, produced inferior stage grouping of early stage cancers (stage 0–IIB squamous cell carcinoma and stage 0–IIA adenocarcinoma) because of inhomogeneity.[6] Superior pathological grouping with improved homogeneity is afforded by the use of *Pathologic Prognostic Groups* and setting the unknown histologic grade or location to X.

Unique TNM categories (ypTisN1-3M0 and ypT0N0-3M0), dissimilar stage group compositions and markedly different survival profiles compared to clinical and pathological staged patients necessitated separate stage groups, identical for both histopathologic cell types, for those patients who have received neoadjuvant therapy (Postneoadjuvant Therapy). UICC failed to list these groups.

Table 4. Post neoadjuvant therapy stage groups (ypTNM) for squamous cell carcinoma and adenocarcinoma*

Stage	T	N	M
Stage I	T0–2	N0	M0
Stage II	T3	N0	M0
Stage IIIA	T0–2	N1	M0
Stage IIIB	T3	N1	M0
	T0–3	N2	M0
	T4a	N0	M0
Stage IVA	T4a	N1–2	M0
	T4a	NX	M0
	T4b	N0-2	M0
	Any T	N3	M0
Stage IVB	Any T	Any N	M1

*Reproduced with permission and adapted from Rice TW, Ishwaran H, Ferguson MK, Blackstone EH, Goldstraw P. Cancer of the esophagus and esophagogastric junction: an 8th edition staging primer. *J Thorac Oncol* 2016; in press.[9]

References

1. Rice TW, Kelsen D, Blackstone EH, Ishwaran H, Patil DT, Bass AJ, Erasmus JJ, Gerdes H, Hofstetter WL. Esophagus and esophagogastric junction. In: Amin MB, Edge SB, Greene FL, et al., eds. *AJCC Cancer Staging Manual*. 8th ed. New York, NY: Springer; 2017:185-202.

2. Oesophagus including oesophagogastric junction. In: Brierley JD, Gospodarowicz MK, Wittekind C, eds. *TNM Classification of Malignant Tumors. International Union Against Cancer*. 8th ed. Oxford, England: Wiley; 2017:57-62.

3. Rice TW, Apperson-Hansen C, DiPaola LM, et al. Worldwide Esophageal Cancer Collaboration: clinical staging data. *Dis Esophagus*.2016;7:707-14.

4. Rice TW, Lerut TEMR, Orringer MB, et al. Worldwide Esophageal Cancer Collaboration: neoadjuvant pathologic staging data. *Dis Esophagus* 2016;7:715-23.

5. Rice TW, Chen L-Q, Hofstetter WL, et al. Worldwide Esophageal Cancer Collaboration: pathologic staging data. *Dis Esophagus* 2016;7:724-33.

6. Rice TW, Ishwaran H, Hofstetter WL, Kelsen DP, Blackstone EH. Recommendations for pathologic staging (pTNM) of cancer of the esophagus and esophagogastric junction for the 8th edition AJCC/UICC staging manuals. *Dis Esophagus* 2016 (in press).

7. Rice TW, Ishwaran H, Kelsen DP, Hofstetter WL, Blackstone EH. Recommendations for neoadjuvant pathologic staging (ypTNM) of cancer of the esophagus and esophagogastric junction for the 8th edition AJCC/UICC staging manuals. *Dis Esophagus* 2016 (in press).

8. Rice TW, Ishwaran H, Blackstone EH, Hofstetter WL, Kelsen DP. Recommendations for clinical staging (cTNM) of cancer of the esophagus and esophagogastric junction for the 8th edition AJCC/UICC staging manuals. Dis Esophagus 2016 (in press).

9. Rice TW, Ishwaran H, Ferguson MK, Blackstone EH, Goldstraw P. Cancer of the esophagus and esophagogastric junction: an 8th edition staging primer. *J Thorac Oncol* 2016 (in press).

21

Site-Specific Explanatory Notes for Carcinoma of the Oesophagus and of the Oesophagogastric Junction

Rules for Classification

The classification applies to all types of carcinoma. Gastrointestinal stromal tumours and neuroendocrine tumours (carcinoids) have their own classifications. The changes in the 8th edition derive from the analyses of the Worldwide Esophageal Cancer Collaboration (WECC).[1-6]

Oesophagus

Summary – Oesophagus (includes oesophagogastric junction)	
T1	Lamina propria, muscularis mucosae (T1a), submucosa (T1b)
T2	Muscularis propria
T3	Adventitia
T4a	Pleura, pericardium, diaphragm
T4b	Aorta, vertebral body, trachea
N1	1-2 regional
N2	3-6 regional
N3	7 or more regional

A tumour the epicentre of which is in the stomach within 5 cm of the oesophagogastric junction and also extends into the oesophagus is classified and staged using the oesophageal scheme. Tumours with an epicentre in the stomach greater than 5 cm from the oesophagogastric junction or those within 5 cm of the oesophagogastric junction without extension in the oesophagus are classified and staged using gastric carcinoma scheme.

There is a proposal to divide carcinomas of the oesophagogastric junction region into three entities:[7-9]

- Adenocarcinoma of the distal oesophagus (AEG I, so-called Barrett carcinoma)
- 'Real' carcinoma of the cardia (AEG II)
- Subcardial carcinoma of the stomach, infiltrating the distal oesophagus (AEG III)

These proposals give some indication of the epidemiology and biology of the tumours. By sampling worldwide data on oesophageal and oesophagogastric junction cancers, it has been shown that patients with all types of Siewert's carcinoma have a similar poor prognosis to patients with oesophageal cancer.[10,11] Therefore, these different types are classified according to tumours of the oesophagus.

The presence of additional synchronous primary carcinomas that are only histologically demonstrable is classified as multifocality and is not considered in the TNM classificaton. For the separation of these carcinomas from skip metastasis (intramural metastasis), the configuration of tumour cells as well as the presence of intraepithelial neoplasia are considered. In contrast to multi-focality, multiplicity, i.e. the presence of additional macroscopically detectable synchronous primary carcinomas is indicated in brackets, e.g. T2(m) or pT2(3).

So-called skip metastasis (intramural metastasis) are tumour foci (orally or abo-rally) separate from the primary carcinoma in the wall of the oesophagus or stomach particularly in the submucosa. Such skip metastasis can be found in 10-15% in oesophageal tumour resection specimen. They are considered the result of lymphatic spread in the oesophageal wall. These 'skip metastasis' are not considered in the TNM/pTNM classification and are not considered metastasis.

Invasion of adventitia (cT3/pT3) corresponds to invasion of perioesophageal soft tissue. This is not considered invasion of the mediastinum or invasion of adjacent structures (T4).

Invasion of pleura, percardium or diaphragm (structures that are usually considered resectable) are classified as T4a.

A carcinoma of the oesophagus that has invaded the stomach and shows a perforation there is classified as pT4a (equivalent to tumours of the stomach). Invasion of bronchi, lung, heart, aorta, V. cava, V. azygos and invasion of recurrent nerve(s) or phrenic or sympathetic nerves (structures that are usually considered unresectable) are classified as T4b.

Invasion in fistulas between oesophagus and trachea or oesophagus and bronchus or compression of V. cava or V. azygos is classified T4b.

Lymph Nodes (Oesophagus)

The definition of the regional lymph nodes of the oesophagus has been simplified in the 7th edition.

The regional lymph nodes, irrespective of the site of the primary tumour, are those in the oesophageal drainage area including coeliac axis nodes and parao-esophageal nodes in the neck.

Paraoesophageal lymph nodes within the neck are considered regional. All other involved lymph nodes above the clavicles (supraclavicular) are classified as distant metastasis.

In the AJCC Cancer Staging Manual 2009 the regional lymph nodes are listed in detail:

Regional Lymph Nodes

Zone	Number	Site
Supraclavicular	1	Supraclavicular
Upper	2	Upper paratracheal
	3p	Posterior mediastinal/upper paraoesophageal
	4 (R, L)	Lower paratracheal (right, left)
AP (aortopulmo-nary)	5	Subaortic aortopulmonary
	6	Anterior mediastinal (anterior to ascending aorta ascendens or innominate artery)
Subcarinal	7	Subcarinal
Lower	8 (L,R)	Middle paraoesophageal (left, right)
	9 (L, R)	Pulmonary ligament (left, right)
Hilar	10 (R, L)	Tracheobronchial (hilar) (right, left)
Thoracal	15	Diaphragmatic
Abdominal	16	Paracardial
	17	Along arteria gastric sinistra
	18	Along arteria hepatica communis
	19	Along arteria lienalis
	20	At the basis of arteria coeliaca

There is a difference in classification of supraclavicular lymph nodes: they are considered as regional in the AJCC Manual, but not in the UICC booklet, where they are designated as distant metastasis.

Another problem arises by the general rule of the TNM system if a tumour involves more than one site or subsite, e.g. contiguous extension to another site or subsite, the regional lymph nodes include those of all involved sites and subsites. According to this rule, all nodes regional for the stomach have to be considered as regional for tumours of the oesophagus and oesophagogastric junction, too. However, in the AJCC list the following stations are missing: perigastric/lesser curvature, perigastric/greater curvature, suprapyloric, infrapyloric, at the splenic hilum.

Stage Grouping and Prognostic Grouping

The T, N and M categories used by the UICC and the AJCC are identical. The UICC presents two options for stage groupings:

1) A purely anatomical approach that applies to all histological types, and
2) A prognostic AJCC approach that has two separate classifications for squamous cell and adenocarcinoma, with the former taking histological grade and subsite into consideration and the latter including histological grade only. The definitions of the prognostic grouping for squamous cell and adenocarcinoma of UICC and AJCC are identical. The AJCC Manual has only the prognostic scheme.

See Chapter 20 for stage grouping and prognostic groups tables.

References

1. Rice TW, Apperson-Hansen C, DiPaola C et al. Worldwide Esophageal Cancer Collaboration: clinical staging data. *Dis Esophagus* 2016;7: 707-14.
2. Rice TW, Chen L-Q, Hofstetter WL et al. Worldwide Esophageal Cancer Collaboration: pathologic staging data. *Dis Esophagus* 2016;7: 724-33.
3. Rice TW, Lerut TEMR, Orringer MB et al. Worldwide Esophageal Cancer Collaboration: neoadjuvant pathologic staging data. *Dis Esophagus* 2016;7: 715-23.
4. Rice TW, Ishwaran H, Hofstetter WL, Kelsen DP, Blackstone EH. Recommendations for pathologic staging (pTNM) of cancer of the esophagus and esophagogastric junction for the 8th edition AJCC/UICC staging manuals. *Dis Esophagus* 2016 (in press).
5. Rice TW, Ishwaran H, Kelsen DP, Hofstetter WL, Blackstone EH. Recommendations for neoadjuvant pathologic staging (ypTNM) of cancer of the esophagus and esophagogastric junction for the 8th edition AJCC/UICC staging manuals. *Dis Esophagus* 2016 (in press).
6. Rice TW, Ishwaran H, Blackstone EH, Hofstetter WL, Kelsen DP. Recommendations for clinical staging (cTNM) of cancer of the esophagus and esophagogastric junction for the 8th edition AJCC/UICC staging manuals. *Dis Esophagus* 2016 (in press).
7. Hermanek P, Henson DE, Hutter RVP, Sobin LH, eds. UICC TNM Supplement 1993. A Commentary on Uniform Use, 1st ed. New York, Wiley; 1993.
8. Sobin LH, Wittekind Ch, eds. UICC TNM Classification of Malignant Tumours, 6th ed. New York, Wiley; 2002.
9. Wittekind Ch, Henson DE, Hutter RVP, Sobin LH, eds. UICC TNM Supplement. A Commentary on Uniform Use, 3rd ed, New York, Wiley; 2003.
10. Rosenberg P, Friederichs J, Schuster T et al. Prognosis of patients with colorectal cancer is associated with lymph node ratio. A single-center analysis of 3026 patients over a 25-year time period. *Ann Surg* 2008; 248: 968-978.
11. Derwinger K, Carlsson G, Gistavsson B. Stage migration in colorectal cancer related to improved lymph node assessment. *Eur J Surg Oncol* 2007; 33: 849-853.

Editorial Addendum

By Thomas W. Rice, MD, and Eugene H. Blackstone, MD

This reprinted manuscript, published in 2012, references material from the UICC 7th edition staging manual. Although some of the material is pertinent today, there are many important changes in the 8th edition.

The Oesophagogastric Junction

The oesophagogastric junction (OGJ) has been redefined for the 8th edition. Use of a simple measurement to define whether a cancer is oesophageal or gastric has impeded OGJ cancer staging since the 1980's. Conflicting statistical analyses necessitated a "place card" consensus decision for the 8th edition. Cancers involving the OGJ that have their epicenter within the proximal 2 cm of the cardia are to be staged as oesophageal cancers. Cancers whose epicenter is more than 2 cm distal from the OGJ, even if the OGJ is involved, will be staged using the stomach cancer TNM and stage groupings.[1] Early work suggests genetic signature of OGJ cancers will be much more useful in appropriate cancer staging by identifying cell of origin rather than relying on gross location.[2,3] A "genetic" definition of the OGJ will obviate the need for further dividing it into thirds (AEG I–III, Siewert I–III). This redefinition of the OGJ will be a focus of the 9th edition staging.

Regional Lymph Nodes

The regional lymph node map has been refined in the 8th edition AJCC staging manual (Figure 22.2).[1] The regional lymph node stations are listed in Table 1. Supraclavicular, perigastric/greater curvature, suprapyloric, infrapyloric, and splenic hilum lymph nodes are non regional lymph nodes in the AJCC 8th edition Cancer Staging Manual.

Stage Grouping and Prognostic Grouping

The recent (7th edition) separation of pathologic groupings into *Pathological Stage* and *Pathological Prognostic Group* by the UICC contradicts the stated purposes of TNM classifications and stage groupings originally set out by the UICC, "Classification is a means of recording facts observed by the clinician whereas staging implies interpretation of these facts regarding prognosis."[4] This superfluous distinction unnecessarily produces confusion and inferior stage grouping (see Chapter 20 Editorial Addendum). With publication of the AJCC 8th edition Cancer Staging Manual and the data-driven placement of oesophageal and OGJ cancers with unknown histologic grade or location the statement "the AJCC manual has only the prognostic scheme" is irrelevant.

References

1. Rice TW, Kelsen D, Blackstone EH, Ishwaran H, Patil DT, Bass AJ, Erasmus JJ, Gerdes H, Hofstetter. Esophagus and esophagogastric junction. In: Amin MB, Edge SB, Greene FL, et al. (Eds.) *AJCC Cancer Staging Manual*. 8th Ed. New York:Springer; 2017:185-202.

2. Cancer Genome Atlas Research Network. Comprehensive molecular characterization of gastric adenocarcinoma. *Nature*. 2014 Sep 11;513:202-9.
3. Hayakawa Y, Sethi N, Sepulveda AR, Bass AJ, Wang TC. Oesophageal adenocarcinoma and gastric cancer: should we mind the gap? *Nat Rev Cancer*. 2016 Apr 26;16:305-18.
4. International Union Against Cancer (UICC). *TNM Classification of Malignant Tumors*. Geneva; 1968.

Table 1. Regional lymph node stations for staging cancer of the oesophagus and oesophagogastric junction

Lymph Node Station	Name	Location
1R	Right lower cervical paratracheal nodes	Between supraclavicular paratracheal space and apex of lung
1L	Left lower cervical paratracheal nodes	Between supraclavicular paratracheal space and apex of lung
2R	Right upper paratracheal nodes	Between intersection of caudal margin of brachiocephalic artery with trachea and apex of lung
2L	Left upper paratracheal nodes	Between top of aortic arch and apex of lung
4R	Right lower paratracheal nodes	Between intersection of caudal margin of brachiocephalic artery with trachea and cephalic border of azygos vein
4L	Left lower paratracheal nodes	Between top of aortic arch and carina
7	Subcarinal nodes	Caudal to carina of trachea
8U	Upper thoracic parae-sophageal lymph nodes	From apex of lung to tracheal bifurcation
8M	Middle thoracic parae-sophageal lymph nodes	From tracheal bifurcation to caudal margin of inferior pulmonary vein
8Lo	Lower thoracic parae-sophageal lymph nodes	From caudal margin of inferior pulmonary vein to oesophagogastric junction
9R	Pulmonary ligament nodes	Within right inferior pulmonary ligament
9L	Pulmonary ligament nodes	Within left inferior pulmonary ligament
15	Diaphragmatic nodes	On dome of diaphragm and adjacent to or behind its crura
16	Paracardial nodes	Immediately adjacent to gastroesophageal junction
17	Left gastric nodes	Along course of left gastric artery
18	Common hepatic nodes	Immediately on proximal common hepatic artery
19	Splenic nodes	Immediately on proximal splenic artery
20	Celiac nodes	At base of celiac artery

Note: Cervical periesophageal level VI and level VII lymph nodes are named as per the head and neck map.

22

Atlas of Oesophagus and of Oesophagogastric Junction Cancer Staging

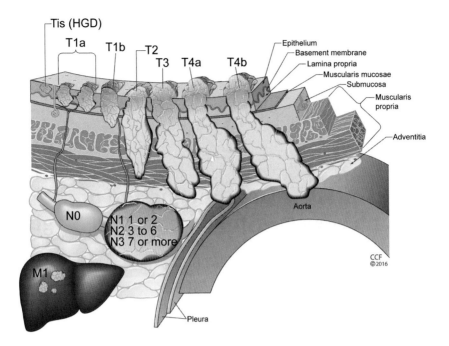

Figure 22.1. Eighth edition TNM categories. T is categorized as Tis: high-grade dysplasia; T1: cancer invades lamina propria, muscularis mucosae, or submucosa and is subcategorized into T1a (cancer invades lamina propria or muscularis mucosae) and T1b (cancer invades submucosa); T2: cancer invades muscularis propria; T3: cancer invades adventitia; T4: cancer invades local structures and is subcategorized as T4a: cancer invades adjacent structures such as pleura, pericardium, azygos vein, diaphragm, or peritoneum and T4b: cancer invades major adjacent structures, such as aorta, vertebral body, or trachea. N is categorized as N0: no regional lymph node metastasis; N1: regional lymph node metastases involving 1 to 2 nodes; N2: regional lymph node metastases involving 3 to 6 nodes; and N3: regional lymph node metastases involving 7 or more nodes. M is categorized as M0: no distant metastasis; and M1: distant metastasis. Copyright ©2016 Cleveland Clinic Foundation, courtesy of Thomas W. Rice, MD.

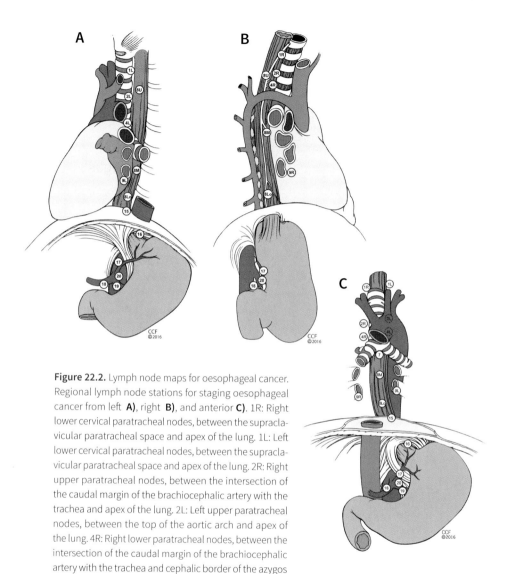

Figure 22.2. Lymph node maps for oesophageal cancer. Regional lymph node stations for staging oesophageal cancer from left **A)**, right **B)**, and anterior **C)**. 1R: Right lower cervical paratracheal nodes, between the supraclavicular paratracheal space and apex of the lung. 1L: Left lower cervical paratracheal nodes, between the supraclavicular paratracheal space and apex of the lung. 2R: Right upper paratracheal nodes, between the intersection of the caudal margin of the brachiocephalic artery with the trachea and apex of the lung. 2L: Left upper paratracheal nodes, between the top of the aortic arch and apex of the lung. 4R: Right lower paratracheal nodes, between the intersection of the caudal margin of the brachiocephalic artery with the trachea and cephalic border of the azygos vein. 4L: Left lower paratracheal nodes, between the top of the aortic arch and the carina. 7: Subcarinal nodes, caudal to the carina of the trachea. 8U: Upper thoracic paraoesophageal lymph nodes, from the apex of the lung to the tracheal bifurcation. 8M: Middle thoracic paraoesophageal lymph nodes, from the tracheal bifurcation to the caudal margin of the inferior pulmonary vein. 8Lo: Lower thoracic paraoesophageal lymph nodes, from the caudal margin of the inferior pulmonary vein to the esophagogastric junction. 9R: Pulmonary ligament nodes, within the right inferior pulmonary ligament. 9L: Pulmonary ligament nodes, within the left inferior pulmonary ligament. 15: Diaphragmatic nodes, lying on the dome of the diaphragm and adjacent to or behind its crura. 16: Paracardial nodes, immediately adjacent to the gastrooesophageal junction. 17: Left gastric nodes, along the course of the left gastric artery. 18: Common hepatic nodes, immediately on the proximal common hepatic artery. 19: Splenic nodes, immediately on the proximal splenic artery. 20: Celiac nodes, at the base of the celiac artery. Cervical perioesophageal level VI and level VII lymph nodes are named as per the head and neck map. Copyright ©2016 Cleveland Clinic Foundation, courtesy of Thomas W. Rice, MD.

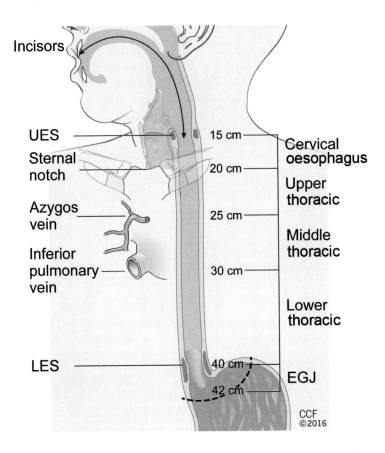

Figure 22.3. Location of oesophageal cancer primary site, including typical endoscopic measurements of each region measured from the incisors. Exact measurements depend on body size and height. Location of cancer primary site is defined by cancer epicenter. Cancers involving the oesophagogastric junction (EGJ) that have their epicenter within the proximal 2 cm of the cardia (Siewert types I/II) are to be staged as oesophageal cancers. Cancers whose epicenter is more than 2 cm distal from the EGJ, even if the EGJ is involved, will be staged using the stomach cancer TNM and stage groups. Key: LES, lower oesophageal sphincter; UES, upper oesophageal sphincter. Copyright ©2016 Cleveland Clinic Foundation, courtesy of Thomas W. Rice, MD.

PART VI

PROGNOSTIC FACTORS

Executive Editor's Note: *It was always recognized that the anatomical extent of disease as described by the TNM classification was not the only prognostic factor. Over the years an increasingly large number of rivals have been recognized; tumor-related, patient-related, environmental factors and, recently, molecular markers. Validation for most of these has been incomplete with few population-based studies of sufficient size to allow multifactorial analysis to assess the confounding impact of other factors. This chapter, contributed by the UICC, summarizes the issues raised by these additional prognostic markers and gives guidance as to future research.*

Acknowledgment: *Used with the permission of the International Union Against Cancer (UICC), Geneva, Switzerland. The original source for this material is in Gospodarowicz MK, O'Sullivan B, Sobin LH, eds. Prognostic Factors in Cancer, 3rd Edition (2006) published by John Wiley & Sons Ltd, www.wiley.com.*

23

Prognostic Factors: Principles and Applications

Mary K. Gospodarowicz, Brian O'Sullivan, and Eng-Siew Koh

Since the beginning of time, humans have wanted to prognosticate, or "know before." In studies of cancer and other diseases, identification of prognostic factors is the present-day equivalent of predicting the future. Nonetheless, it would be implausible to believe that we can predict precisely for the individual patient. In reality, all we can provide are statements of probability, and even these are more accurate for groups of patients, the study of whom provides us with our knowledge about prognosis. The practical management of cancer patients requires us to make predictions and decisions for individuals, and the challenge of prognostication is to link the individual patient to the collective population of patients with the same disease. The rationale for prognostic factors and classifications of these factors with attention to those used in this book are outlined below. The potential endpoints relevant to oncology, the taxonomy of prognostic factors, and their applications in practice and, most importantly, a concept of a management scenario that forms the basis for defining prognosis at a given point in the course of disease, are presented. The "management scenario" is defined within a specific setting, since prognosis differs for different situations, taking account of the therapeutic milieu, the features of the host and disease, and the particular outcome under study. Prognostic factor research, like clinical trials, must observe essential principles of study assembly and analysis if meaningful conclusions are to be drawn.

Rationale for Prognostic Factors

The management of patients, or clinical practice, has four main components. Three comprise actions: namely, diagnosis, treatment, and prevention, and one is advisory, that of prognosis. Appraisal of a patient's prognosis is part of every-day practice, and studies of prognostic factors are integral to cancer research. To consider management of an individual cancer case, the fundamental pieces of information required include the site of origin (e.g., lung or breast), and morphologic type or histology (e.g., adenocarcinoma or squamous cell carcinoma).[1-4] In addition, the outcome in a cancer patient depends on a variety of variables referred to as prognostic factors. These factors are defined as variables that can account for some of the heterogeneity associated with the expected course and outcome of a disease. Knowledge of prognostic factors helps us to understand the natural history of cancer. The range of applications for prognostic factors is outlined in Table 23.1.

Classifications of Prognostic Factors

There are well-defined and accepted classifications of diseases that include cancer. The best known is ICDO, widely used by cancer registries and administrative bodies. The World Health Organization (WHO) Classification of Tumors forms the basis for the histologic classification in cancer. The TNM classifications published by the International Union Against Cancer (UICC) and the American Joint Committee on Cancer (AJCC) are the standard system for recording anatomic disease extent. In contrast to these evidence- and consensus-based agreements, these is no consensus on the optimal classification of prognostic factors. Although no formal system for classifying prognostic factors exists, numerous prognostic indexes and nomograms have been successfully implemented in clinical practice. Previously, we proposed an extremely simple framework for describing prognostic factors in cancer,[2,5] which included the subject-based classification developed to highlight the

Table 23.1. Application of Prognostic Factors: Learning about the Natural History of Disease.

Patient Care

- Select appropriate diagnostic tests
- Select an appropriate treatment plan
- Predict the outcome for individual patient
- Establish informed consent
- Assess the outcome of therapeutic intervention
- Select appropriate follow-up monitoring
- Provide patient and caregiver education

Research

- Improve the efficiency of research design and data analysis
- Enhance the confidence of prediction
- Demarcate phenomena for scientific explanation
- Design future studies
- Identify subgroups with poor outcomes for experimental therapy
- Identify groups with excellent outcomes for simplified therapy
- Identify candidates for organ preservation trials

Cancer Control Programs

- Plan resource requirements
- Assess the impact of screening programs
- Introduce and monitor clinical-practice guidelines
- Monitor results
- Provide public education
- Explain variation in the observed outcomes

importance of nontumor related prognostic factors, and clinical relevance classification to highlight the factors indispensable for good clinical practice.

Subject-Based Classification

Most cancer literature equates prognosis with tumor characteristics. Examples include histologic type, grade, depth of invasion, or the presence of lymph-node metastasis. Cancer pathology and anatomic disease extent account for most variations in cancer outcome. However, factors not directly related to the tumor also affect the course of disease and the outcomes of interest. To consider all prognostic factors, we proposed three broad groupings that will be developed further in this edition: those factors that relate to disease or tumor, those that relate to the host or patient, and those that relate to the environment in which we find the patient. In this edition, we focus on prognostic factors that are relevant at the time of diagnosis and initial treatment, although in the management of cancer patients, determination of prognosis is required repeatedly at multiple situations along the course of the disease. These situations often reflect decision-making points, for example, about adjuvant therapy, management of recurrent cancer, and palliative or terminal care.

Tumor-Related Prognostic Factors.
These include those directly related to the presence of the tumor or its effect on the host, and most commonly comprise those that reflect tumor pathology, anatomic disease extent, or tumor biology (Table 23.2). The fundamental factor to consider is definition of a particular cancer as a distinct disease entity. While histology forms the basis of tumor classification today, the recent revolution in molecular

Table 23.2 Examples of Tumor-Related Prognostic Factors

1. **Pathology**
   Molecular tumor characteristics; gene expression patterns
   Morphologic classification (e.g., adenocarcinoma, squamous)
   Histologic grade
   Growth pattern (e.g., papillary vs. solid, cribriform vs. tubular, vs. solid)
   Pattern of invasion (e.g., perineural, small vessel invasion)

2. **Anatomic tumor extent**
   TNM categories
   Tumor bulk
   Single versus multifocal tumor
   Number of sites of involvement
   Tumor markers (e.g., PSA, AFP, CEA)

3. **Tumor biology**
   Tumor markers (e.g., HER2-neu, CD20)
   Proliferation indices (e.g., S-phase fraction, MiB-1)
   Molecular markers (p53, rb, Bcl2)

4. **Symptoms (related to the presence of tumor)**
   Weight loss
   Pain
   Edema
   Fever

5. **Performance status**

medicine has challenged today's classification and has led to redefinition of many cancers according to molecular and genetic tumor characteristics. These newer criteria have been now accepted in acute leukemia and subtypes of lymphoma. Most new tumor-related molecular factors, such as gene expression patterns, deal with disease characterization.

The second fundamental group of prognostic factors relate to the anatomic extent of disease, so-called "stage," classified according to the UICC TNM classification.[6] In addition to the TNM categories and stage groupings, factors describing disease extent, including tumor bulk, number of involved sites, or involvement of specific organs, and tumor histology, also have an impact on prognosis.[7-10]

Tumor pathology is crucial to the determination of prognosis in cancer. The histologic type has traditionally defined the disease under consideration, but additional factors, such as grade, pattern of growth, immunophenotype, and more recently gene expression patterns, also reflect the fundamental type of disease under consideration. In contrast, multifocality, presence of lymphatic or vascular invasion, infiltration patterns that also affect the outcome may relate both to type of disease and the extent.[11,12] Tumor markers like prostatic-specific antigen (PSA), alpha-feto protein (AFP), and beta human chorionic gonadotropin (HCG) are used in everyday practice and strongly correlate with tumor bulk.[13-15] Hormone receptors, biochemical markers, expression of proliferation-related factors and, increasingly, molecular tumor characteristics that have been shown to affect outcomes for a variety of cancers relate to the type of cancer.[16-18] The presence of symptoms has generally been considered a host factor but it may also be a tumor related factor. A classic example is the presence of B-symptoms (night sweats, fever, and weight loss) in Hodgkin lymphoma.

Host-Related Prognostic Factors. These are factors present in the body of the host (patient) that are not directly related to malignancy, but through interference with the behavior of the tumor or their effect on treatment have the potential to significantly impact the outcome. These factors may generally be divided in demographic patient characteristics, such as age,[19] gender,[20] and racial origin,[21] comorbidity and coexistent illness,[22,23] especially those affecting the immune status,[24] performance status related to comorbid illness, and factors that relate to the host mental state, attitude, and compliance[25,26] with therapy. A history of prior cancer and treatment of that cancer also places survivors at risk for future events (Table 23.3).

Environment-Related Prognostic Factors. The factors that operate external to the patient and could be specific either to an individual patient or, more frequently, to groups of patients residing in the same geographic area. Here, we can consider three categories of environmental factors: first, those that have a physician expertise focus, such as the choice of a specific treatment plan and caregiver skill; second a healthcare system focus including access[27,28] to cancer care, caliber of medical record keeping, internet access,[29] degree of clinical trial participation, and also the presence of ageism, which can all influence treatment selection and outcome. Finally, there are factors related to a society focus, such as a patient's socioeconomic,[30] and nutritional status, and the overall quality of care, including the presence of quality control programs,[31] which may impact the outcome (Table 23.4).

While a classification within the three subject-based categories may be a useful working model, the distinction between these groupings of prognostic factors is not always clear and many prognostic factors overlap these categories. For example, performance status may be related to the tumor, or, when compromised due to coexistent illness, could be a host-

Table 23.3. Examples of Host-Related Prognostic Factors

1. Demographics
Age
Race
Gender
Level of education
Socioeconomic status
Religion

2. Comorbidity
Constant
  – Inherited immune deficiency
  – von Recklinghausen disease, etc.
Changeable
  – Coexistent illness
    (e.g., inflammatory bowel disease, collagen vascular disease)
  – Weight
  – Cardiac status
  – Acquired immune deficiency
  – Infection
  – Mental health

3. Performance status

4. Compliance
Social reaction to illness
Influence of habits, drugs, alcohol, smoking, etc.
Belief in alternative therapies

related prognostic factor. Similarly, the quality of treatment is a host-related factor if it relates to patient compliance, but is usually an environment-related factor relating to access to optimal medical care. An example of a prognostic factor that fits into all the subject-based categories is anemia[32] and all three could apply to the same patient. Anemia may be a direct result of the presence of tumor mass, as in superficial bladder cancer or cervix uteri cancer, because of persistent heavy bleeding. It may also be a host factor, as in a patient with thalassemia or anemia of chronic disease from an unrelated condition. However, in some parts of the world, as an environmental prognostic factor, anemia also may be a result of malnutrition.

Several prognostic factors, each individually giving predictions with relatively low accuracy, can be combined to provide a single variable of high accuracy. Such a variable is called a prognostic index. Other examples include the International Lymphoma Prognostic Index (IPI)[33] or the Eastern Cooperative Oncology Group (ECOG) performance status scale.

Table 23.4. Examples of of Environment Related Prognostic Factors.

	Related to		
	Treatment	**Education**	**Quality**
Physician	Choice of physician or specialty • Quality of diagnosis • Accuracy of staging Choice of treatment Expertise of physician, "narrow experts" Timeliness of treatment Ageism	Ignorance of medical profession Access to internet Knowledge, education of the patient Participation in clinical trials Participation in continuing education	Quality of treatment Skill of the physician Treatment verification
Health Care System	Access to appropriate diagnostic methods Access to care • Distance • Waiting lists • Monopoly control of access to care Availability of publicly funded screening programs	Continuing medical education Lack of audit of local results Access to internet Development of practice guidelines Dissemination of new knowledge	Quality of equipment Quality management in treatment facility Maintenance of health records Availability of universal health insurance Quality of diagnostic services Implementation of screening programs Promotion of error free environment
Society	Preference for unconventional therapies Socioeconomic status Distance from cancer center Insurance status Access to transportation, car, etc. Ageism	Literacy Access to information	Access to affordable health insurance Nutritional status of the population

Clinical-Relevance-Based Classification

To consider the relevance of prognostic factors in clinical practice, prognostic factors in this book are placed in three distinct categories: essential, additional, and new and promising factors. Essential factors are those that are fundamental to decisions about the goals and choice of treatment, and include details regarding the selection of treatment modality and specific interventions. In this edition, we have asked the authors to classify as essential exclusively those factors that are required to meet a published clinical practice guideline. This was not possible in all the cases, and as for the other parameters, some variation in the interpretation of the proposed additional factors allow finer prognostication, but are not an absolute requirement for treatment related decision-making processes. Their role is to communicate prognosis, but they do not in themselves influence treatment choice. Finally, our new and promising factors are those that shed new light about the biology of disease, or the prognosis for patients, but for which currently there is, at best, incomplete evidence of an independent effect on outcome or prognosis.

Essential Prognostic Factors. The fundamental factors required to make treatment decision is the type of cancer defined by histology or molecular tumor characteristics. The second most important group of essential factors reflects the anatomic disease extent. The latter has been recognized for over 75 years, when the first attempts at staging classifications were made. Currently, the UICC TNM6 and the AJCC[34] serve to facilitate worldwide communication about cancer. Many other essential factors have been identified including pathology, tumor biology, tumor-related symptoms, patient age, performance status, newer imaging methods,[35-37] and tumor markers[38] are also integral to the decision-making process in the choice of a treatment modality.

Additional Prognostic Factors. In addition to the essential factors, there are numerous variables that help to define the outcome more precisely, but are not required for general decisions about treatment. These include more detailed histologic features, host-related factors, including comorbid conditions and vital organ function, which influence the suitability for surgery, chemotherapy, or radiotherapy. Environment-related factors, such as the choice of an inferior treatment plan, poor quality diagnostic tests, or treatments themselves have the potential to compromise the outcome. Management in a specialized unit,[39] for example, in breast and colorectal cancer, has resulted in improved survival in population-based studies.

New and Promising Prognostic Factors. The immense and rapid expansion of molecular biology has provided an abundance of opportunities to study new biologic prognostic factors,[40,41] which hold promise for future applications. Molecular factors, such as epidermal growth factor receptor (EGFR) status,[42,43] may be used to predict response to a treatment modality, or may present a target for therapy, such as imatinib in gastrointestinal stromal tumors.[44] Alternatively, they may assist in treatment stratification, such as MGMT status, which predicts for chemotherapy and radiotherapy responsiveness in glioblastoma multiforme.[45] Another category includes factors that predict for the presence of occult distant metastases.

A combination of the subject-based and clinical-relevance-based classifications can be used to summarize in simple terms the prognostic factors for individual cancers for a selected management scenario, as depicted in Table 23.5.

Table 23.5. Examples of Prognostic Factors in Cancer.

Prognostic Factors	Tumor Related	Host Related	Environment Related
Essential	Anatomic disease extent Histologic type	Age	Availability of access to a radiotherapy facility
Additional	Tumor bulk Tumor marker level	Race Gender Cardiac function	Expertise of a surgeon
New and promising	EGFR (lung, head and neck) Gene expression patterns	Germline p53 mutation	Access to information

Management Scenarios: Freezing the Prognosis

Since prognosis is a dynamic process affected not only by time, but also other factors, such as the disease and intervention, it is thus useful to apply the concept of *management scenario*, which freezes the prognostic attributes that exist at a given time point, enabling one to then consider how prognosis is influenced by the choice of the planned intervention and the outcome of interest (Figure 23.1).

For example, in *scenario 1* during a normal physical examination prior to lumpectomy, a patient is found to have a 2-cm breast cancer. Considering the overall survival as the outcome of interest, her prognosis equates to that of reported survival for clinical stage I breast cancer in her peer group (age, race, socioeconomic status) and in geographic region. After the initial treatment is completed, the patient is in *scenario 2*. She has a pTl pNO tumor. Her prognosis is better than in scenario 1. She elects to be managed with partial mastectomy alone, her prognosis in scenario 2 is thus less favorable for local control than if she chose to have adjuvant radiation therapy. However, her prognosis for overall survival may not be affected by this decision. After some time, we can construct *scenario 3*. Thus, some years later she develops local recurrence and distant metastasis (scenario 3). Her prognosis for survival is now much worse than in previous scenarios. The progress of time may also affect positively the probability of survival.

Since the prognosis differs with a given scenario, prognostic factors should be considered within a given context or scenario, most commonly before a definitive treatment plan is formulated. Since treatment interventions also have a major impact on the outcome, it is important to discuss prognostic factors in the context of a specific treatment plan or therapeutic intervention.

Endpoints Relevant to Consider in Cancer Patients

The relevant endpoints to consider in cancer include probability of cure, duration of survival, likelihood of response to treatment, probability of relapse, time to relapse, likelihood of local tumor control, likelihood of organ preservation, and possibility for symptom relief in a palliative context.[46] Therefore, the outcomes may be very heterogeneous. Moreover, some prognostic factors facilitate prediction of more than one outcome, while others predict selected outcomes only.

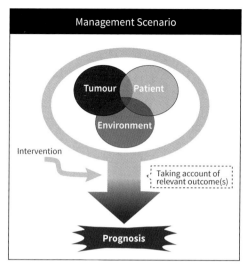

Figure 23.1. Representation of the interaction among the three domains of prognostic factors (tumor, host, and environment). The prognostic factors are expressed in the context of the proposed therapeutic intervention and for a given endpoint of interest (e.g., survival, response, local tumor control, organ preservation). In addition, the prognosis itself must be interpreted in the context of both the treatment (because it may change the prognosis) and the endpoint (which must be relevant to the prognosis).

For example, the presence of bladder muscle wall invasion by a transitional cell carcinoma predicts for distant failure, while its absence virtually eliminates this probability. This knowledge permits clinicians to ignore the possibility of distant failure in patients with superficial bladder cancer both in diagnostic tests and therapeutic interventions. Another example is the number of involved nodal regions in stages I and II Hodgkin's disease that predict for risk of treatment failure, but not for survival. The number of tumors in superficial bladder cancer is predictive for recurrence, but has no impact on the overall survival.

Response to Treatment and Prognosis. Response to treatment is an outcome and as such it always reflects the prognosis. If a response to treatment had no impact on the outcome, such treatment by definition would be ineffective. However, since the knowledge of response is not available until after treatment is initiated, response should not be considered a prognostic factor for the scenario that preceded it.

Tumor response is an early endpoint in the assessment of treatment effectiveness. The four categories of response (complete response, partial response, stable disease, and progressive disease) were originally proposed by the World Health

Organization (WHO).[47] Although initially developed to assess the effects of drug therapy, these same criteria may easily be applied to the outcomes of surgical or radiotherapy interventions. For example, complete tumor resection with negative margins could be considered as a complete response to surgical intervention, while positive resection margins could be considered as a partial response to surgical intervention. Thus the extent of response is a surrogate for the anatomic extent of disease after the completion of therapy, and as such is a prognostic factor for further outcome. Since the knowledge of response is not available until after treatment is completed, it should not be considered a prognostic factor for the scenario that preceded it.

Taxonomy: Prognostic Factors

In the English language, prediction, forecasting, and prognosis all indicate the probability of future events. In medical literature, however, the use of the terms, such as predictive, prognostic, and risk are being freely substituted for each other without much thought about consistent and accurate definitions.

In 1994, Burke[50] proposed that the general heading of predictive factors describe three subtypes: a risk, a diagnostic, and a prognostic factor. In his definition, a risk factor was a factor where the main outcome of interest was incidence and the predictive accuracy was <100%; the diagnostic factor was where the outcome of interest was the incidence and the predictive accuracy was almost 100% of disease. A prognostic factor was where the outcome of interest was death and the predictive accuracy was variable. This classification did not consider the temporal attributes of prediction and is associated with too narrow a view of relevant endpoint for patients with cancer. In epidemiological literature, a risk factor is defined as "a clearly defined occurrence or characteristic that has been associated with the increased rate of a subsequently occurring disease"; thus it is limited to patients who currently do not have a disease. In contrast, a prognostic factor refers to a probability of future event in patients who do currently have a disease.

Henderson and Patek[51] and others defined the term "predictive" as "prognosis for a measurable response" of overt tumor reduction following a treatment intervention and used the term "predictive factor" as distinct from "prognostic" factor. The authors then consider a prognostic factor in the narrow context of a probability of cure or prolongation of survival. An example of a prognostic factor that is not a predictive factor is the number of involved axillary lymph nodes in breast cancer.[8] A high number of lymph nodes is associated with inferior survival, but the number of involved lymph nodes has no impact on response to treatment. In contrast, a factor that is both predictive and prognostic is the estrogen receptor status in breast cancer that predicts for response to hormonal therapy, but also prognosticates for a better survival. It is debatable whether such a distinction in terminology, which focuses on a single intermediate outcome (a measurable response to cytotoxic treatment) instead of defined endpoint relating to overall prognosis (e.g., local tumor control, survival), should be embraced.

Examples of clinical situations where response is not an indication for the use of treatment include: chemotherapy in an asymptomatic patient with Stage III follicular small-cell lymphoma; androgen deprivation therapy in an asymptomatic patient with Tl prostate cancer; and radiation therapy in stage IV Hodgkin's lymphoma.

Surrogate Diagnostic Factors versus Prognostic Factors. With better understanding of the mechanisms by which prognostic factors predict the future, new endpoints other than long-term survival have emerged. For example, the forecasting of the probability of occult distant metastasis allows for a better understanding of the pattern of failure and targeting of treatment efforts. Where the probability of the presence of occult metastatic disease at the time of diagnosis is concerned, however, these factors predict for the current state and not for a future event. Two examples of such factors are the PSA level[13] and the Gleason score in localized prostate cancer, which are considered as prognostic when survival or treatment failure probabilities are the endpoints of interest, but seen as surrogate diagnostic factors when they help discriminate different states at the present time. The reason is that they may help determine the probability of the presence of subclinical disease (e.g., disease lymph-node involvement) as an endpoint of interest.

Time-Dependent Prognostic Factors. Time-dependent prognostic factors are variables that become available over the time course of the patient's disease. While they may be very predictive of outcome, they are also problematic because they risk disturbing the context of relevant disease outcome evaluation and decision making.[52] This is because it may be impossible to separate real "causality" in the relationship between a time-dependent factor and an outcome of interest from a mere "association" caused by another factor common to them both. Therefore, if not undertaken carefully, the clinical interpretation of time-dependent prognostic factors may be incorrect. In some cases, prognostic factors associated with a subsequent scenario have been considered together with prognostic factors at diagnosis. For example, the postradiotherapy PSA nadir level has been included in Cox models of prognostic factors in localized prostate cancer. In truth, the PSA nadir is a surrogate for response to radiotherapy,[13] and as such belongs to a different management scenario occurring subsequently.

Application of Prognostic Factors

Prognostic factors are used in daily clinical practice, in research, and in cancer control. In everyday clinical practice, the influence of prognostic factors dominates all the steps in decision making and the comprehensive management of patients with cancer, including selection of the primary goal of management, the most appropriate treatment modality, and the adjustment of treatment according to disease severity. Knowledge of prognostic factors allows clinicians to select treatment options that allow preservation of organs or function without compromising cure and survival.

The implementation of evidence-based clinical practice guidelines[53] will also serve to improve the quality of decision making and in turn the outcomes in cancer patients. It is thus necessary to know the prognostic factors in a relevant context in order to evaluate compliance with such guidelines to then examine their impact.

Prognostic Factors and Milieu

The prognostic factors that are defined as essential for decision making depend on their relevance to the issues in cancer care in a particular milieu, that is, the practice of cancer care in the first world or conversely in developing countries,[54] where the main issues are related to cancer prevention and early detection. Factors that predict for organ preservation and those that contribute to finesse in defining the prognosis may not be important in places with limited diagnostic equipment, and where funding for evaluation of assessment of response to treatment is not available. The milieu where the patient and health care professional are located thus impacts on the interplay of essential, additional, and new and promising factors. Moreover, progress in such situations does not require new discovery, but rather economic development, education, and a continued process to ensure improved access.

Future Research into Prognostic Factors

To be relevant to the clinical practice, prognostic factors must either have a significant impact on cancer outcome, or be used to select treatment methods. It is likely that with progress in treatment, and improved outcomes, prognostic factors will be more relevant for selection of treatment. However, knowledge of prognostic factors is also required to minimize the impact of treatment. Improved staging methods, and especially more accurate characterization of microscopic disease extent will allow a more homogeneous grouping of patients with similar disease characteristics, and the tumor-related prognostic factors for an individual disease may change. Knowledge of genetic factors will further add to the improved prediction of outcome and greater individualization of therapeutic interventions. However, grouping of patients into similar categories will continue to be required to assess the impact of new technology of patient assessment and new therapies on the outcome.

References

1. Byar D: Identification of prognostic factors, in Buyse ME SM, Sylvester RJ (eds.): Cancer clinical trials. New York: Oxford University Press, 1984, pp. 423-443.

2. Gospodarowicz M, O'Sullivan B: Prognostic Factors: Principles and Application, in Gospodarowicz M, Henson DE, Hutter RVP, et al. (eds.): Prognostic Factors in Cancer. 2nd ed. New York; Wiley-Liss, 2001, pp. 17-36.

3. Stockier M, Tannock I: Guide to studies of diagnostic tests, prognostic factors, and treatments, in Tannock I, Hill, R. (eds.): The basic science of oncology, 3rd ed. Toronto; McGraw-Hill, 1998, pp. 466-492.

4. Riley RD, Abrams KR, Sutton AJ, et al.: Reporting of prognostic markers: current problems and development of guidelines for evidence-based practice in the future. *Br J Cancer* 88:1191-1198,2003.

5. Gospodarowicz M, O'Sullivan, B, Bristow, et al.: Host, and Environment-related Prognostic Factors, in Gospodarowicz M, Henson DE, Hutter RVP et al. (eds.): Prognostic Factors in Cancer, 2nd ed. New York; Wiley-Liss, 2001, pp. 71-94.

6. Sobin LH, Wittekind C: TNM classification of malignant tumors. 6th ed. New York; Wiley-Liss, 2002.

7. Schmoll HI, Souchon R, Krege S, et al.: European consensus on diagnosis and treatment of germ cell cancer: a report of the European Germ Cell Cancer Consensus Group (EGCCCG), *Ann Oncol* l5:1377-1399, 2004.

8. Truong PT, Berthelet E, Lee I, et al.: The prognostic significance of the percentage of positive/dissected axillary lymph nodes in breast cancer recurrence and survival in patients with one to three positive axillary lymph nodes. *Cancer* 103:2006-2014, 2005.

9. Compton CC: Colorectal carcinoma: diagnostic, prognostic, and molecular features. *Mod Pathol* l6:376-388,2003.

10. Berglund M, Thunberg U, Amini RM, et al.: Evaluation of immunophenotype in diffuse large B-cell lymphoma and its impact on prognosis. *Mod Pathol* l8:1113-1120, 2005.

11. Baak IP, van Diest PI, Voorhorst FI, et al.: Prospective multcenter validation of the independent prognostic value of the mitotic activity index in lymph node-negative breast cancer patients younger than 55 years. *J Clin Oncol* 23:5993-6001, 2005.

12. Truong PT, Yong CM, Abnousi F, et al.: Lymphovascular invasion is associated with reduced locoregional control and survival in women with node-negative breast cancer treated with mastectomy and systemic therapy. *J Am Coll Surg* 200:912-921, 2005.

13. D'Amico AV, Renshaw AA, Sussman B, et al.: Pretreatment PSA velocity and risk of death from prostate cancer following external beam radiation therapy. *JAMA* 294:440-447, 2005.

14. Gorog D, Regoly-Merei I, Paku S, et al.: Alpha-fetoprotein expression is a potential prognostic marker in hepatocellular carcinoma. *World J Gastroenterol* 11:5015-5018, 2005.

15. Paramasivam S, Tripcony L, Crandon A, et al.: Prognostic importance of preoperative CA-125 in International Federation of Gynecology and Obstetrics stage I epithelial ovarian cancer: an Australian multicenter study. *J Clin Oncol* 23:5938-5942, 2005.

16. DiGiovanna MP, Stem DF, Edgerton SM, et al.: Relationship of epidermal growth factor receptor expression to ErbB-2 signaling activity and prognosis in breast cancer patients. *J Clin Oncol* 23:1152-1160, 2005.

17. Wang Y, Klijn IG, Zhang Y, et al.: Gene-expression profiles to predict distant metastasis of lymph-node-negative primary breast cancer. *Lancet* 365:671-679, 2005.

18. Buscarini M, Quek ML, Gill P, et al.: Molecular prognostic factors in bladder cancer. *RIU Int* 95:739-742, 2005.

19. HurriaA, Leung D, Trainor K, et al.: Factors influencing treatment patterns of breast cancer patients age 75 and older. *Crit Rev Oncol Hematol* 46:121-126, 2003.

20. Batevik R, Grong K, Segadal L, et al.: The female gender has a positive effect on survival independent of background life expectancy following surgical resection of primary non small cell lung cancer: a study of absolute and relative survival over 15 years. *Lung Cancer* 47:173-181, 2005.

21. Chlebowski RT, Chen Z, Anderson GL, et al.: Ethnicity and breast cancer: factors influencing differences in incidence and outcome. *J Natl Cancer Inst* 97:439-448, 2005.

22. Maas HA, Kruitwagen RF, Lemmens VE, et al.: The influence of age and co-morbidity on treatment and prognosis of ovarian cancer: a population-based study. *Gynecol Oncol* 97:104-109,2005.

23. Janssen-Heijnen ML, van Spronsen DI, Lemmens VE, et al.: A population-based study of severity of comorbidity among patients with non-Hodgkin's lymphoma: prognostic impact independent of International Prognostic Index. *Br J Haematol* 129:597-606, 2005.

24. Straus DJ: Prognostic factors in the treatment of human immunodeficiency virus associated non-Hodgkin's lymphoma. *Recent Results Cancer Res* 159: 143-148, 2002.

25. Verkooijen HM, Fioretta GM, Rapiti E, et al.: Patients' refusal of surgery strongly impairs breast cancer survival. *Ann Surg* 242:276-280, 2005.

26. Cathcart CS, DunicanA, Halpern IN: Patterns of delivery of radiation therapy in an innercity population of head and neck cancer patients: an analysis of compliance and end results. *J Med* 28:275-284, 1997.

27. Mackillop WJ, Zhang-Salomons J, Groome PA, et al.: Socioeconomic status and cancer survival in Ontario. *J Clin Oncol* 15:1680-1689, 1997.

28. Jemal A, Ward E, Wu X, et al.: Geographic patterns of prostate cancer mortality and variations in access to medical care in the United States. *Cancer Epidemiol Biomarkers Prev* 14:590-595,2005.

29. Till JE, Phillips RA, Jadad AR: Finding Canadian cancer clinical trials on the Internet: an exploratory evaluation of online resources. *CMAJ* 168: 1127-1129, 2003.

30. Freeman HP: Poverty, culture, and social injustice: determinants of cancer disparities. *CA Cancer J Clin* 54:72-77, 2004.

31. Sauven P, Bishop H, Patnick J, et al.: The National Health Service Breast Screening Programme and British Association of Surgical Oncology audit of quality assurance in breast screening 1996-2001. *Br J Surg* 90:82-87, 2003.

32. Munstedt K, Johnson P, Bohlmann MK, et al.: Adjuvant radiotherapy in carcinomas of the uterine cervix: the prognostic value of hemoglobin levels. *Int J Gynecol Cancer* 15:285-291, 2005.

33. Hermans J, Krol AD, van Groningen K, et al.: International Prognostic Index for aggressive non-Hodgkin's lymphoma is valid for all malignancy grades. *Blood* 86:1460-1463,1995.

34. AJCC Cancer Staging Manual. 6th ed.: Springer-Verlag, 2002.

35. Borst GR, Belderbos JS, Boellaard R, et al.: Standardised FDG uptake: a prognostic factor for inoperable non-small cell lung cancer. *Eur J Cancer* 41:1533-1541, 2005.

36. Hutchings M, Mikhaeel NG, Fields PA, et al.: Prognostic value of interim FDG-PET after two or three cycles of chemotherapy in Hodgkin lymphoma. *Ann Oncol* 16: 1160-1168, 2005.

37. Jackson AS, Parker CC, Norman AR, et al.: Tumor staging using magnetic resonance imaging in clinically localised prostate cancer: relationship to biochemical outcome after neo-adjuvant androgen deprivation and radical radiotherapy. *Clin Oncol* (R Coll Radiol)17: 167-171,2005.

38. Lam JS, Shvarts 0, Leppert JT, et al.: Renal cell carcinoma 2005: new frontiers in staging, prognostication and targeted molecular therapy. *J Urol* 173:1853-1862, 2005.

39. Smith ER, Butler WE, Barker FG, 2nd: Craniotomy for resection of pediatric brain tumors in the United States, 1988 to 2000: effects of provider caseloads and progressive centralization and specialization of care. *Neurosurgery* 54:553-563; discussion 56 3-555, 2004.

40. Poon RT, Fan ST, Wong J: Clinical significance of angiogenesis in gastrointestinal cancers: a target for novel prognostic and therapeutic approaches. *Ann Surg* 238:9-28, 2003.

41. Russo A, Bazan V, Iacopetta B, et al.: The TP53 Colorectal Cancer International Collaborative Study on the Prognostic and Predictive Significance of p53 Mutation: Influence of Tumor Site, Type of Mutation, and Adjuvant Treatment. *J Clin Oncol* 23:7518-7528, 2005.

42. Shepherd FA, Rodrigues Pereira J, Ciuleanu T, et al.: Erlotinib in previously treated non small-cell lung cancer. *N Engl J Med* 353:123-132, 2005.

43. Bentzen SM, Atasoy BM, Daley FM, et al.: Epidermal growth factor receptor expression in pretreatment biopsies from head and neck squamous cell carcinoma as a predictive factor for a benefit from accelerated radiation therapy in a randomized controlled trial. *J Clin Oncol* 23:5560-5567, 2005.

44. Van Glabbeke M, Verweij J, Casali PG, et al.: Initial and late resistance to imatinib in advanced gastrointestinal stromal tumors are predicted by different prognostic factors: a European Organisation for Research and Treatment of Cancer-Italian Sarcoma Group-Australasian Gastrointestinal Trials Group study. *J Clin Oncol* 23:5795-5804, 2005.

45. Hegi ME, Diserens AC, Gorlia T, et al.: MGMT gene silencing and benefit from temozolomide in glioblastoma. *N Engl J Med* 352:997-1003, 2005.

46. Toscani P, Brunelli C, Miccinesi G, et al.: Predicting survival in terminal cancer patients: clinical observation or quality-of-life evaluation? *Palliat Med* 19:220-227, 2005.

47. WHO handbook for reporting results of cancer treatment, Geneva: World Health Organization Offset Publication, 1979.

48. Zagars GK, Ballo MT, Pisters PW, et al.: Surgical margins and reresection in the management of patients with soft tissue sarcoma using conservative surgery and radiation therapy. *Cancer* 97:2544-2553, 2003.

49. Smitt MC, Nowels K, Carlson RW, et al.: Predictors of reexcision findings and recurrence after breast conservation. *Int J Radiat Oncol Biol Phys* 57:979-985, 2003.

50. Burke HB: Increasing the power of surrogate endpoint biomarkers: the aggregation of predictive factors. *J Cell Biochem Suppl* 19:278-282, 1994.

51. Henderson IC, Patek AJ: The relationship between prognostic and predictive factors in the management of breast cancer. *Breast Cancer Res Treat* 52:261-288, 1998.

52. McShane LM, Altman DG, Sauerbrei W, et al.: Reporting recommendations for tumor marker prognostic studies (REMARK). *J Natl Cancer Inst* 97: II 80-II 84, 2005.

53. Woolf SH: Evidence-based medicine and practice guidelines: an overview. *Cancer Control* 7:362-367, 2000.

54. Magrath I, Shanta V, Advani S, et al.: Treatment of acute lymphoblastic leukaemia in countries with limited resources; lessons from use of a single protocol in India over a twenty year period. *Eur J Cancer* 41:1570-1583, 2005.

24

Developing a Prognostic Prediction Model for Lung Cancer

Frank Detterbeck

"It is highly desirable for the physician to apply himself
diligently to the art of foreshadowing" –Hippocrates

There is no question that there is a strong desire in medicine to predict prognosis, particularly when dealing with patients with cancer. While most people have an intuitive general sense about prognosis, we would like to be more scientific. However, it has been difficult to achieve a solid scientific basis for doing so. Despite a plethora of papers specifically addressing prognostic factors in lung cancer, no reliable, validated prognostic prediction model for this disease has emerged. The vast majority of papers claim positive results, but have used flawed methods that provide overly optimistic results and most have lacked further validation.[1,2]

However, major advances have been made in understanding what constitutes scientifically sound research in prediction modeling. We need to apply this knowledge in order to meet the needs of patients and physicians. This chapter examines concepts and challenges related to prognostic prediction, with the goal of achieving a deeper level of understanding that may help define strategies to develop tools to predict prognosis moving forward. The focus is on patients with lung cancer, and on outcomes generally considered most relevant for patients with cancer.

This chapter addresses prognostic prediction models–it does not discuss the preliminary step of identifying potential prognostic factors. Prognostic factor studies can be classified as phase I (exploring a potential association between a possible factor and a surrogate for outcome), phase II (exploring an association between a possible factor and outcomes) and phase III (confirmatory studies in well-defined patients demonstrating that a marker is associated with good or poor outcomes).[3] This is different from using prognostic factors to build a model (that accounts for the degree of prognostic value as well as that of other factors) to predict outcomes in patients.

What Do We Want from a Prognostic Model?

A starting point is to reflect on what the actual goals are that are meant to be fulfilled by a prognostic model. At the most basic level is the innate human desire to know what the future holds, an age-old desire that has been the basis for interpreters of horoscopes, tea leaves and palm readers for ages. More concretely, we wish to know what is the chance of cure or the duration of survival of a patient. Inherent in this statement are the desires to make a prediction for a specific individual, and to define the actual outcome. This information can be useful to guide decisions about how to prioritize various aspects of a person's ongoing life.

Estimating prognosis quickly becomes intertwined with predicting outcomes associated with a specific treatment approach (or no treatment). Because treatment approaches change over time as advancements are made, this highlights how fluid the nature of prognostic prediction is. In addition, a clinically relevant prognostic prediction model should apply to present day patients; we want to use what we have learned from past experiences to be able to make predictions for present patients about their outcomes in the future. Finally, we want a prognostic prediction that applies to an individual patient, not an average outcome of a patient population.

Fundamental Concepts Regarding Prognostic Prediction

Prognostic prediction is an inherently different process than classification (e.g. stage classification of patients with lung cancer).[4] Stage classification is fundamentally a nomenclature that enables clear communication about the anatomic extent of a tumor. A nomenclature must remain stable (with only periodic refinement). It must be able to be applied consistently, so that everyone classifies a particular tumor the same way (given the same information, e.g. imaging or biopsy results). Stage classification is a statement of a fact regarding a particular tumor. Prognostic prediction, however, refers to a guess about what will happen to a patient. It is inherently speculative (about future outcomes) and associated with a degree of uncertainty. It is fluid and constantly changing as treatments evolve and depending on the management. The prognosis of different individuals with tumors of the same stage is not necessarily the same, and the prognosis of the same individual (with the same tumor) in different settings will be different. While tumor stage impacts a patient's prognosis, and observed prognosis is used as a tool to decide upon a classification system, stage classification and prediction of prognosis remain fundamentally different processes.

Prognosis of a patient with cancer depends on many different factors. These can be grouped into 3 major domains: tumor-related, patient-related and environment-related (Figure 24.1). Within each of these domains there are many individual factors that may be important. In addition, the prognosis depends on the clinical scenario (the treatment given or planned, the point in time relative to the diagnosis or treatment etc.). Finally, it also depends on the outcome of interest (overall survival, disease-specific survival, recurrence, treatment response, toxicity, quality of life etc.).

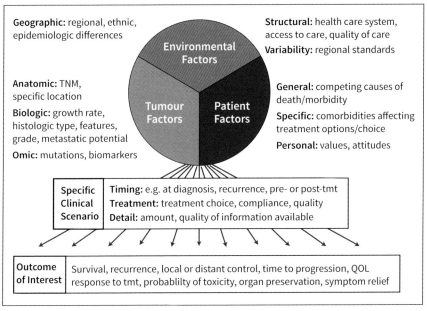

Figure 24.1. Schematic of Domains of Prognostic Factors. Omic, genomic, transcriptomic, proteomic, metabolomic factors; QOL, quality of life; tmt, treatment

Both the actual and relative impact of a particular prognostic factor often depend on other prognostic factors and on the clinical scenario. For example, for a patient with advanced stage small cell lung cancer (SCLC) the impact of co-morbidities or environmental factors is likely to be minimal, whereas for a patient who has successfully completed curative intent treatment of a stage IA non- small cell lung cancer (NSCLC) survival is likely to be determined primarily by patient-related and environmental factors and less by tumor-related factors. Another example is that the actual impact of an Epidermal Growth Factor Receptor (EGFR) mutation is dramatically different whether the patient is being considered for treatment with an EGFR inhibitor or not.

Technically, a prognostic factor is one that inherently influences the outcome of patients regardless of (any) treatment(s) received, whereas a predictive factor is one that predicts a response to a particular treatment (Table 24.1).[5] While this

Table 24.1. Glossary of Terms

Term	Description	Specific Measures or Examples
Prognostic factor	A factor associated with an outcome regardless of any treatment	Stage, age (for overall survival)
Predictive factor	A factor that predicts that a treatment effect will occur (or not)	EGFR mutation (for treatment with an EGFR inhibitor)
Event	Outcome of interest. From a statistical viewpoint, it is the smaller of either events or non-events that determines the power to evaluate variables	Absence of death (overall survival), Absence of death from the disease of interest (Disease-Specific Survival); Death from the disease of interest (Disease-specific mortality)
Dichotomization	The process of splitting a continuous variable into 2 groups. While this provides results that are conceptually easier to grasp, it is discouraged because information is thrown away, and how the split is done can affect validity	Age < vs ≥65; size < vs ≥4 cm
Calibration	How close is the agreement between the outcome prediction from the model and the observed outcome?	Calibration plot (observed on y-axis vs predicted on x-axis)
	Intercept assesses a systematic, consistent shift	Intercept (also known as alpha or calibration-in-the-large
	Slope assesses the agreement relative to the spectrum of outcomes	Slope (also known as beta); e.g. better performance in higher risk patients
Discrimination	How well does the model correctly predict a good or bad outcome between pairs of individuals	C-index, D-statistic, area under ROC curve
Overall performance measures	Overall statistical assessment of model performance	Explained variation (R^2), Brier score,
Internal validation	Techniques applied using the study cohort to adjust for overfitting (i.e. an overly optimistic assessment of the model's performance)	Bootstrapping, cross validation; (split sample, apparent performance are discouraged)
External validation	Assessment of model performance in an independent (external) patient cohort	
Reproducibility	Assessment in an independent cohort that is nearly the same as the model development cohort	This demonstrates generalizability in the same population

Transport-ability	Assessment in an independent cohort that is similar yet different (e.g. setting, time period, region)	This demonstrates broad generalizability
Risk grouping	The process of simplifying a prediction model by splitting patients into risk groups. Groups should be defined by clinical (not statistical) considerations	Details of how groups and cutpoints are chosen is critical for validity
Classification measures	Measures to assess how often the model correctly places a patient into a risk group. (Often this implies that the risk group thresholds have relevance for clinical management which has not been demonstrated)	Predictive value, sensitivity, specificity
Decision curve analysis	A decision curve depicts how altering a threshold for a decision making affects the net benefit of the model (the model's false positive and false negative rate)	

EGFR, epidermal growth factor receptor; ROC, receiver operating characteristic

distinction is useful in some situations, it is questionable whether this distinction can really be made in the context of a prognostic prediction model. There is little clinical relevance to a prediction in the absence of treatment. If we want to have a prediction for actual patients that are going to be treated in some manner, factors that have an impact are essential regardless of whether they are prognostic or predictive.

If a prognostic model is to meet clinical needs, the endpoint of the model should be chosen thoughtfully. This depends on the intended use of the model and the clinical scenario. A major differentiation is whether the patient is eligible for curative-intent treatment vs palliative treatment, as the outcomes of interest and their relative importance differ. For curatively treatable patients, the chance of cure is perhaps more relevant than overall survival (OS) that includes all causes of death. This specific focus raises the importance of disease-specific survival (with either recurrence or death due to the disease being endpoints) rather than disease free survival (with either recurrence or death from any cause counting as an event). A short-term treatment-related impairment of quality of life is likely to be less important if the chance of cure is high. However, long-term quality of life (relative to a non-disease related baseline) remains very important. Unfortunately, cause of death data is less available, and recurrence is affected by the follow-up policy.

For patients who are treated palliatively, the length of anticipated survival is likely to be important (i.e. median, or survival at a particular point such as

12 months). The quality of life is very important, and a measure that represents both the duration and the quality of life may be ideal. How this is best defined from a patient's perspective is unclear.

It is crucial to be clear about the starting point for an estimate of prognosis as this dramatically influences the estimate; as patients progress through time multiple starting points are relevant (in fact, essentially a continuum). In using an estimate to guide decisions about treatment, the obvious starting point is before treatment (after the evaluation to define the clinical stage is finished). As an aid to set priorities in a patient's life, multiple points are valuable: before treatment, after successful (or not) completion of treatment, at various subsequent time points (e.g. 6, 12, 24 months after completion), either with or without a recurrence.

Status of Prognostic Modeling for Lung Cancer in 2016
Brief Overview of Prognostic Prediction Models in Lung Cancer to Date

The AJCC recently undertook a systematic review of prognostic models in lung cancer intended for clinical use.[1] Of the 32 prognostic tools identified, 25 involved NSCLC and 7 SCLC. The quality of these tools was disappointing. How prognostic factors were selected for analysis was generally not reported, and papers frequently focused on particular new factors without inclusion of established, readily available factors. Only 17% used robust internal validation methods; most used "apparent" internal validation techniques that led to overly optimistic estimates of the model's predictive ability. Few models assessed calibration or discrimination; most erroneously assumed that statistically significant differences between risk groups provided an assessment of internal validity. External validity in an independent dataset was evaluated in one third, but only 6%, 16% and 13% externally evaluated calibration, discrimination or overall performance, respectively, with an appropriate method (percentages are not additive because some studies performed several of these assessments).[1]

A recent systematic review of potential protein biomarkers identified by immunohistochemistry (IHC) in NSCLC from 2008-13 found that robust identification of such factors is still at a fledgling level.[6] This study included 347 papers and involved 342 proteins. Almost 40% of the studies involved <100 patients and although 64% of studies reported a marker that was significant by multivariate analysis, only 26 proteins showed consistent prognostic association in ≥2 independent cohorts. The study also confirmed findings on previously (before 2008) identified proteins: Ki67 and NKX2-1 correlated with outcome in most studies, whereas the impact of EGFR, Cyclin D1 and TP53 is inconsistent and questionable. Use of a panel of markers is similar, with no panel available that shows independent predictive power.[6]

Prognostic gene-expression signatures have also been extensively investigated. This is a complex field, and many details of the design, genetic testing and statistical analysis are crucial. The potential pitfall of erroneously identifying a "prognostic factor" due to overfitting (overly optimistic assessment) is tremendously magnified in genomic, transcriptomic and proteomic studies, in which the number of variables is much larger than the number of patients. This is poignantly illustrated by Subramanian et al.:[7] using an actual cohort of 129 patients and 5000 random gene profiles, many impressive "prognostic factors" (i.e. >3-fold difference in OS, p < 0.001) were able to be identified purely at random in a training set (which all failed to show any prognostic value in an internal split validation set).[7]

These reviews indicate that the quality of studies addressing prognostic factors in lung cancer is low. The studies are primarily exploratory investigations that are hypothesis-generating about potential prognostic factors, but require further evaluation before they can be used clinically (see next section). Several other reviews (both of lung cancer as well as cancer in general) also have identified widespread issues related to quality of both the reporting and the design of studies, which seriously limit the ability of the studies to advance the science.[2,8-13] Particular weaknesses to highlight are use of a retrospective convenience sample, poor accounting for other characteristics (e.g. age, stage, treatment), use of re-substitution statistics (first defining an optimal cutpoint, then assessing statistical significance),[14] lack of appropriate tests to assess incremental predictive power over conventional prognostic factors (e.g. concordance statistic or other measures), poor reporting (of patients, design, methods) that prevents validation and lack of appropriate internal and external validation. The poor quality of the studies and reporting persists despite the establishment of reporting criteria for tumor marker studies (REMARK) in 2005.[15]

Only a few prognostic prediction models for lung cancer have undergone external validation (Table 24.2). Liang et al recently published a prognostic model for OS in R0 resected early stage NSCLC patients.[16] This study was well designed and reported (addressing almost all of the Transparent Reporting of a multivariable prediction model for Individual Prognosis or Diagnosis [TRIPOD] standards),[17,18] involved an appropriately large patient cohort and included external validation in a large and broad cohort (from the IASLC 1999-2010 dataset). The factors identified and included in the final model were age, sex, histology, number of nodes sampled, pT and pN stage. The calibration and discrimination of the model were high in both the internal and external validation set.

In association with the 7th edition stage classification, the International Association for the Study of Lung Cancer (IASLC) Staging and Prognostic Factors Committee (SPFC) developed a model in resected NSCLC patients and validated this against similar patients in the SEER database.[19] The large size of the development cohort and the detailed analysis as well as the fact that it holds up in a large validation assessment with regional and temporal differences makes this a strong

Table 24.2. Selected Prognostic Models for Lung Cancer.

1st Author (year)	% met of TRIPOD Criteria[a]	Level of Evidence	Population	N Patients (events)	End-point	Model Method	Model type	Internal Validation Methods	External Validation Methods	N Patients (events)	Factors Identified
Liang[16] (2015)	79%	2-narrow validation	Resected NSCLC	5,261 (1,746)	OS	Cox, AIC	Nomogram, Risk groups	Bootstrap, C index, calibration	C index, calibration	2,148 (762)	Age, sex, histology, NNS, T, N
Chansky[19] (2009)	61%	3-broad validation	Resected NSCLC	9,137 (?)	OS	Cox, RPA	RPA	bootstrap	Survival curves	9,221 (?)	Age, sex, p-stage
Dehing-Oberije[21] (2009)	65%	2-narrow validation[b]	ChRT for cI-IIIB NSCLC	322 (?)	OS	2-norm vectors, ROC	Nomogram, Risk groups	bootstrap	ROC	101 (?)	sex, PS, FEV1, GTV, no. of + node stations
Mandrekar[22] (2006)	81%	2-narrow validation	cIIIB-IV NSCLC	782 (?)	OS	Cox	equation, grid of subgroups	bootstrap	subgroup calibration	426 (?)	PS, age, Hgb, WBC
Non-Validated Models											
Zhang[23] (2014)	79%	1-development	Advanced NSCLC	773 (700)	OS	Cox, ROC	tertile	Bootstrap, split sample	none	—	Age, stage, surgery, chemotherapy, drinking, Alb, INR, Prot, BUN, ALP
Okayama[25,26] (2014)	61%	1-development	Resected pI adeno	817 (?)	OS	Cox	Nomogram, Risk groups	—	none	—	4-Gene risk group, pIA vs IB, age, sex
Dehing-Oberije[20] (2011)	67%	1-development	ChRT for cI-IIIB NSCLC	106 (71)	OS	2-norm vectors, ROC	Nomogram, Risk groups	bootstrap	internally split sample[c]	—	sex, PS, FEV1, GTV, no. of + node stations, CEA, IL-6

Models are included that have been externally validated or meeting a high quality level of reporting. [a]Studies did not explicitly or deliberately follow the TRIPOD standards, [b]including a separate report; [c]refined model validated in a temporally split internal validation set; not counted as external validation due to the cohorts were small and temporally and regionally very similar to development cohort limited difference in time periods (May 2004 to May 2006 vs June 2006 to November 2007).

Adeno, adenocarcinoma; AIC, Akaike Information Criterion; Alb, albumin; Alp, alkaline phosphatase; BUN, blood urea nitrogen; CEA, carcinoembryonic antigen; ChRT, treated with Chemoradiotherapy; FEV1, forced expiratory volume in 1 second; GTV, gross tumor volume; Hgb, hemoglobin; IL-6, Interleukin 6; INR, international normalized ratio; NNS, number of nodes sampled, NSCLC, Non-small cell lung cancer; OS, overall survival; Prot, serum protein level; PS, performance status; ROC, receiver operating characteristic curve; RPA, recursive partitioning and amalgamation; TRIPOD, Transparent Reporting of a multivariable prediction model for Individual Prognosis or Diagnosis standards; WBC, white blood cell count;

model. However, the detail of the reporting and the assessment method for the validation does not correspond to what is currently viewed as appropriately robust.

A model was developed by Dehing-Oberjie et al to predict 2-year OS in patients with stage cI-IIIB NSCLC treated with chemoradiotherapy 2002-6.[20] All patients were staged with PET and CT; about 20% were stage I and ~70% stage IIIA,B. All traditional prognostic factors were assessed (age, sex, PS, comorbidity, weight loss, T, N, stage, histology, number of node stations involved, tumor volume and treatment). The model was externally validated in 3 independent cohorts of Dutch patients; the AUC for the ROC curves for the development and 3 validation sets were 0.74, 0.75, 0.79 and 0.72, respectively.[20,21] However, each of the validation cohorts had far fewer than the recommended number of events (i.e. 100-200) and involved cohorts that are regionally and temporally closely related to the development cohort, making the validation rather weak. This model was later refined to include CEA and IL-6 blood levels after evaluation of 8 potential blood biomarkers, but this new model has only been weakly validated in an small internally split sample.[20]

The North Central Cancer Treatment Group pooled results of 9 treatment trials in stage IIIB-IV NSCLC from 1985 through 2003 to develop a model for OS, which was validated in a 1996-98 trial cohort.[22] The final model included age, performance status (PS), and hemoglobin and white blood cell counts, selected from a many standard laboratory values and patient- and tumor-related factors. The model development was very carefully done. The validation focused on calibration, but the report left out discrimination and details that limit the assessment of the model's performance.

A few non-validated prognostic prediction models deserve mention. Zhang et al. developed a model for stage IIIB and IV (7th Edition) NSCLC that used readily available laboratory measures, clinical and tumor related variables to predict OS (Table 24.2).[23] The quality of the report itself was very high. Unfortunately, the study suffers from a major flaw because performance status data was not available. Furthermore, only split-sample internal validation was done.[23] This model identified factors that are different than other larger models in a similar population,[22,24] highlighting the difficulties associated with developing models that are ready for clinical use.

A recent model focused on the use of gene expression to prognostically classify resected stage I adenocarcinoma.[25,26] The final model included stage (pIA vs IB), age and a 4-gene classifier. These genes were chosen from a list of genes likely to have prognostic value from preclinical studies, and the 4-gene classifier was validated in multiple (11) independent cohorts. The prognostic prediction model itself was not validated, but the quality and thoroughness of evaluating and validating the 4-gene classifier as a prognostic factor is a strength of this model. Shortcomings include that the number of events is inherently low (typical of stage I), and that the cohorts, although multiple and geographically and temporally diverse, represent a convenience sample for which tissue was available. A hurdle for implementation is that the assessment requires fresh-frozen tissue. Nevertheless, the thoroughness of evaluation of the 4-gene classifier makes this model promising, if confirmed in external validation.

Other recent models are not discussed because they were not externally validated and had shortcomings in how they were developed or reported that hinder further refinement or validation (i.e. addressing only a minority of the TRIPOD criteria),[27-30] or represent studies to identify prognostic factors rather than develop a model.[24]

Quality Standards for Prognostic Modeling

Standards for appropriate derivation, reporting and validation of prognostic models have long been established. Formal standards for the derivation of a prognostic model, developed by the Evidence-Based Medicine Working Group, were published in *JAMA* in 2000 (Table 24.3).[31] This article also contains standards for external validation and criteria that should be met in order for a prognostic model to be considered ready for clinical use (Table 24.4). These standards have endured, being consistently adopted in subsequent standards that have focused primarily on how studies should be reported (Table 24.5). The most recent standards for reporting prognostic model studies (TRIPOD)[17,18] involves a 22 point reporting checklist, and an extensive detailed description of nuances and options (to use or not to use) that raise the quality of reporting. These standards are based on a systematic review, solid science, and were developed by an international expert team in an extensive 3 year formal process.[17,18]

It is surprising that the general quality of prognostic modelling studies is so poor (corresponding to the lowest level of evidence in Table 24.4), despite the long history of well publicized, consistent standards. Most likely, this is because adhering to the demands of good science as summarized in these standards is not easy. It requires a large enough and detailed enough database, sophisticated techniques and extensive validation. The temptation is great to

Table 24.3. Methodological Standards for Derivation of a Prognostic Model for Clinical Use

1. Were all important predictors included in the derivation process?
2. Were all important predictors present in a significant proportion of the study population?
3. Were all the outcome events and predictors clearly defined?
4. Were those assessing the outcome event blinded to the presence of the predictors and those assessing the predictors blinded to the outcome event?
5. Was the sample size adequate (meaning adequate number of outcome events)?
6. Does the model make clinical sense?

Taken from McGinn et al. User's Guide to the Medical Literature XXII: How to Use Articles About Clinical Decision Rules[31]

Table 24.4. Levels of Evidence to Guide the Use of Prediction Models.

Level of Evidence	Definition and Standards of Evaluation	Implications for Use
1. Derivation of prediction model	Identification of predictors using multivariate model; blinded assessment of outcomes	Needs validation and further evaluation before using clinically in actual patient care
2. Narrow validation of prediction model	Verification of predictors when tested prospectively in 1 setting; blinded assessment of outcomes	Needs validation in varied settings; may use predictors cautiously in patients similar to sample studied
3. Broad validation of prediction model	Verification of predictive model in varied settings with wide spectrum of patients and physicians	Needs impact analysis; may use predictions with confidence in their accuracy
4. Narrow impact analysis of prediction model used as decision model	Prospective demonstration in 1 setting that use of prediction model improves physicians' decision (quality or cost-effectiveness of care)	May use cautiously to inform decisions in settings similar to that studied
5. Broad impact analysis of prediction model used as decision model	Prospective demonstration in varied settings that use of prediction model improves physicians' decisions for wide spectrum of patients	May use in varied settings with confidence that its use will benefit patient care quality or effectiveness

Adapted from Reilly et al.58 and the Evidence-Based Medicine Working Group[31]

publish a finding based on a small sample size, showing impressively separated survival curves – albeit using flawed statistics that provide an overly optimistic assessment. A common misconception is that merely finding statistical significance in multivariate analysis demonstrates the usefulness of a prognostic model; this is clearly not true. If journals adhere to the existing reporting standards the number of publications will diminish drastically. However, given how little progress has been made in lung cancer to establish robust prediction models despite the plethora of publications, a decrease in number with an increase in scientific rigor would be a positive development.

Many advances have been made in the statistical development and assessment of prognostic models. A few points are highlighted. With regard to model development it is crucial that the patients, the outcomes and the factors under consideration are clearly defined. It is critical that standard prognostic factors (e.g. stage, age, performance status) be included in the analysis. The number of events (the lowest of either those with or without the outcome in question) is what matters, not the number of patients. A traditional rule of thumb has been that the sample should be large enough to yield at least 10 events per variable (EPV),[32-34] but recent data[35] suggest that ≥20 EPV are needed to generate model performance measures that are sufficiently stable when subjected to external validation. For internal

Table 24.5. Formal Standards Regarding Prognostic Models.

Acronym	Year	Title	Description
User's Guide[31]	2000	User's Guides to the Medical Literature XXII: How to Use Articles About Clinical Decision Rules	Standards for derivation, external validation, and when to consider a prognostic model appropriate for clinical application
REMARK[15]	2005	REporting for tumor MARKer prognostic studies	Describes aspects that should be reported; specifically addresses tissue studies
STREGA[45]	2009	STrengthening the REporting of Genetic Association/Studies – An Extension of the STROBE Statement	Focuses on details and specific to consider and report in genetic association studies
GRIPS[43,44]	2011	Strengthening the reporting of Genetic RIsk Prediction Studies	This follows closely the design and statistical reporting standards for prognostic models in general and has little regarding specifics for genomic studies
CHARMS[59]	2014	Critical Appraisal and Data Extraction for Systematic Reviews of Prediction Modelling Studies	Criteria for reporting and critical evaluation of systematic reviews of prognostic modeling studies
TRIPOD[17]	2015	Transparent Reporting of a multivariable prediction model for Individual Prognosis or Diagnosis	Detailed description of what should be reported

validation, splitting into a training and validation set is inefficient and should be avoided (unless the sample size is very large).[17,35] Bootstrapping (or cross-validation) is recommended, producing only a small degree of optimism compared with external validation (at least 200 bootstrap samples).[17,35,36]

External validation samples need to be sufficiently large to have reasonable power to detect relevant differences (e.g. 80% power to detect a performance 1.5 times too high or too low or a difference of ≥ 0.1 in the area under a receiver operating characteristic [ROC] curve). Several studies have demonstrated that the validation sample should have a minimum of 100-200 events.[17,37,38] An appropriate assessment should include evaluating discrimination (e.g. c-index, ROC curve, D statistic), calibration (e.g. graphic, intercept & slope), and overall performance (e.g. R^2, Brier score).[17,37,39] If the external cohort is very similar to the development cohort, the performance assessment is one of reproducibility; however if the cohort is similar but with some differences (e.g. different time period, different clinical setting) it provides a measure of transportability. Recently, a statistical method has been proposed to quantify the degree of similarity between the development and a validation cohorts and thus aid the interpretation of external validation studies.[40]

In addition to the statistical issues associated with model development and assessment, there are many technical issues associated with biomarkers (e.g. genetic markers or IHC). Formal, widely accepted standards for IHC analyses are not available. A recent article discusses many technical details involved and suggests standards to be followed.[41] A 7-step guide to validating an antibody is also provided in another publication.[42]

Studies involving gene alterations pose a particular problem due to the multitude of alterations. Methods to avoid overly optimistic results have been developed, with a number of different approaches being appropriate depending on the nature of the question and the data at hand; there is no single correct way to structure a study. Quality standards for reporting genetic prognostic factors have been developed[43-45] and approaches to this area of research that provide a more realistic assessment of prognostic value have been defined.[11]

An additional issue in lung cancer is that the most prominent genetic biomarkers are primarily predictive factors applicable to the specific scenario of receiving targeted therapy.[46] Their overall prognostic impact outside of this scenario is less well defined. Developing a model that includes very specific treatment scenarios, or allows for different effects of genetic markers in different clinical scenarios is very complex. Therefore, this remains a difficult area.

The AJCC has recently identified acceptance criteria for prognostic models (Table 24.6).[47] The SPFC encourages research into prognostic modeling, but these must have a solid scientific and statistical basis before they can be taken seriously. The criteria outlined in Table 24.6 provide a reasonable framework for researchers.

Issues Regarding Development of a Prognostic Prediction Model from a Mature Dataset

A model must be based on data; this requires a strong mature dataset. An appropriate dataset must contain a large enough collective of patients (and events). It should include data on all major factors that are known or suspected to have a major impact on prognosis (without many missing data elements). If major known factors are missing, the model prediction may be misleading. Appropriate statistical methods, as outlined previously, must be used to develop the model.

In order to be interpreted appropriately, the prediction provided by a model must have a measure of the degree of uncertainty (e.g. confidence intervals). Techniques are available to accomplish this, and this should be part of the statistical development of a good model. In addition, there is another layer of inherent uncertainty when one considers that there is variability in how well most prognostic factors can be assessed. What type of imaging or biopsies were involved in defining the T, N and M? How standardized and reproducible is the test, for example, of a biomarker? Ideally the model would include generally observed variability in

Table 24.6. AJCC Acceptance Criteria for Prognostic Prediction Models.

Inclusion Criteria (all must be fulfilled)

1. The predicted outcome must be overall survival (OS), disease-specific survival (DSS) or disease-specific mortality (DSM). Other endpoints (e.g. progression, recurrence) involve additional complexities (e.g. definitions, assessment frequency), preventing inclusion at this time.
2. The model should address a clinically relevant question.
3. "Standard" factors should be addressed (i.e. factors that most clinicians would expect to see in the particular context, e.g. age, stage, performance status). It is acceptable if such factors are explicitly considered but justifiably removed (e.g. due to lack of incremental predictive ability)
4. The model should precisely identify the characteristics of the patients used for the development and validation process (e.g. inclusion/exclusion criteria).
5. Generalizability and external validation should be assessed including reproducibility and transportability (i.e. applicability to somewhat different patient populations).
6. The starting point for the model (time zero) should be clearly defined (e.g. at diagnosis, after treatment).
7. All predictors must be known and sufficiently defined at the time zero of the model.
8. The model detail must be made available (e.g. the equation) or open access must be made available (e.g. on a website)
9. A measure of discrimination must be reported (e.g. concordance index).
10. Predicted probability vs observed outcome must be provided (i.e. calibration in the small).
11. The model should be validated in a time frame and setting (e.g. treatment, diagnostic and patient evaluation process) that is relevant to contemporary patients.
12. It should be clear which initial treatment(s) were applied. The model needs not be restricted to a specific treatment, but how patient in the development and validation set were treated should be reported).
13. The model must be published in a peer-reviewed journal.

Exclusion Criteria (if any one is present)

1. A substantial proportion of patients in the validation set are lacking follow-up information (either missing or too short).
2. No information is available regarding missing values in the validation set.
3. The number of events in the validation set is small (e.g. <100)

Taken from Kattan et al.[47]

assessing the prognostic factors in an assessment of uncertainty. But the user must also consider how one's local setting may differ from the general setting in which the model was derived.

At one extreme, a model can be constructed from a large population, using simple, widely available factors (e.g. T, N, M, age, sex). Such a dataset is typically larger and more readily available (both for model development and external validation). However, the prediction essentially applies only to another such population as a whole. It is questionably applicable for a patient that is exactly the average of the population used for model derivation. This is because most factors cannot be defined as an average (except perhaps age). What represents an average sex, an average race, an average treatment? If assessment of the effect of such parameters was not included in the model development, we cannot be sure of how the model actually functions for specific categories of patients. At the opposite extreme, a model that includes tremendous detail, and thus might provide a more accurate prognosis for a patient with matching characteristics, suffers from other challenges. The availability of datasets with such detail is limited. The number of scenarios for which a model must be developed (and validated) becomes challenging. More complex models with multiple variables tend to be overfitted,[48] and smaller sample size for model development will lower the model's performance when applied in an independent cohort.

The number of different factors, specific cohorts and scenarios in which they may (or not) have prognostic significance escalates rapidly. For example, an Epidermal Growth Factor Receptor (EGFR) mutation is highly prognostic in the setting of advanced disease if the patient is to be treated with an EGFR inhibitor; if any of these points do not apply, the prognostic value is reduced. The relationship of a factor may be simple (linear) or require use of a complex function.

Having an all-encompassing, complete and detailed database is probably unrealistic, although coming as close to this as possible is essential. Researchers are encouraged to carry out studies that identify prognostic factors and/or develop models, as long as they involve adequate scientific rigor and adhere to reporting standards. These can help identify prognostic factors that are consistently significant, and can provide an understanding of how they perform in different settings and subgroups.

We need to develop tools and criteria that allow us to combine the predictive power of a factor as defined in one dataset to another. The ability to define when this can reasonably be done (or not) is important to make use of the entirety of well-done research. Most importantly, however, this would provide a basis for flexibility and an ability to appropriately include future factors that are not currently recognized. Being transparent and explicit about the uncertainty associated with an estimate of prognosis provides a mechanism to deal with statistically problematic issues brought about by practical realities, such as finding reasonably appropriate ways to combine data from different studies.

Issues Regarding Prospective Estimation of Prognosis

A model derived from a mature (historic) dataset defines the outcome that a hypothetical patient would have experienced if he/she had been diagnosed during the time period of the retrospective database and in a similar setting. That is not a very clinically relevant measure. We want to estimate outcomes for patients encountered today, not for a hypothetical patient diagnosed and managed in an earlier time period.

Making a prediction for patients cared for in the present about their future outcome, i.e. prospective estimation of prognosis, involves several challenges beyond that of a retrospective prediction model. There has been a marked improvement of prognosis over time (about 30-100%, stage for stage, comparing the IASLC 1990-1999 vs the 1999-2010 dataset).[49] Therefore, any prediction based on past experience must be appropriately adjusted to reflect such a progression. There is inherent uncertainty in estimating how an outcome such as survival will evolve. Some factors driving this may progress linearly, but others may have a more stepwise effect. This may involve particular subgroups of patients differently (e.g. the impact of PET on stage III and IV NSCLC[50-53] or discovery of a targeted therapy for a specific subgroups of patients). Tools to project anticipated general changes over time need to be developed. To quote Winston Churchill: "it is difficult to make predictions, especially about the future".

An external validation (e.g. temporal or regional) may show a systematic shift in all predictions (i.e. systematically altering calibration in one direction without altering the model's discrimination), or may reveal more complex discrepancies compared with the development data. Adjustments to the model can be made through a process of model updating.[17,54,55] There are many levels of complexity that this can involve, ranging from an overall single adjustment of the baseline risk (calibration intercept), inclusion of an overall single adjustment of regression coefficients as well (calibration slope), additional factor-specific adjustments of regression coefficients, addition of new prognostic factors into the model, re-estimation of the entire model using the combined development and validation data (without or with the addition of new prognostic factors).[17] It is controversial whether and to what degree such adjustments are acceptable without representing essentially a new model that must undergo external validation once again before being appropriate for clinical use.[17,39,54-56]

Especially for predictions that are meant to apply to present patients we need to provide a measure of uncertainty together with any estimate of prognosis. Because future predictions are inherently speculative, assessment of the uncertainty is not a purely quantitative (statistical) undertaking. Methods to usefully express this uncertainty need to be developed.

Issues Regarding Individualized Estimation of Prognosis

What physicians (and patients) want, ideally, is a prediction that is tailored for a specific individual patient. This level of detail makes model development much more complex. Furthermore, conventional statistical descriptions of uncertainty describe how random cohorts (samples) of similar patients will fit with the estimate (e.g. a 95% confidence interval indicates that 95% of random additional samples will have an outcome that will fall within this range). Such confidence intervals do not indicate that 95% of an *individual patient's outcome* will fall within this range.

The more individualized an estimate of prognosis is, the more difficult it becomes to be accurate and confident about the prediction.[57] On a group level, one can account for the average rate of occurrence of random events (e.g. being hit by a bus), but this becomes more difficult on an individual level. This is akin to the philosophical difficulty in understanding what a partial outcome (e.g. a 30% 5-year survival)—i.e. a measure designed for a cohort—means when applied to an individual patient.

Issues Regarding Implementation of a Clinically Relevant Model

While appropriate internal validation (e.g. bootstrapping) can adjust for overfitting (making the model seem better than it actually is), a model must be independently validated before it can be trusted and considered for clinical use is selected settings (level 2 evidence, Table 24.4). Ideally, the model should be validated in multiple independent datasets composed of a spectrum of patients and settings to demonstrate broad applicability (level 3 evidence). More ideal yet would be to have an impact study demonstrating that use of the model to guide clinical management (e.g. whether to administer adjuvant chemotherapy) actually achieves the intended effect (level 4 evidence). An estimate of prognosis by itself does not guarantee that appropriate management decisions will be made, or that any treatment intervention will actually make a difference.

Accomplishing these higher levels of evidence represents a major, perhaps unrealistic, challenge when one considers the number of patients and the follow-up needed together with the complexity, pace of change and fluidity that a clinically relevant model should have. Surrogate measures that are more easily accomplished than the formal evaluations mentioned are needed. However, at the very least a single external validation (in another mature dataset that captures past experience) is needed before a model can be suggested to be put to clinical use.

A clinically relevant prognostic prediction model should apply to individuals in the present. It is inherently problematic to apply a retrospective model to the future (as opposed to testing how well it works in another retrospective cohort). One issue is that while we want to have a robust scientific basis for what we do, there is inherently no way to test or validate how well a model works in present patients (until these patients have become part of a retrospective cohort). Furthermore, once we are able to define prognosis for an individual or group of people, we immediately set out to try to improve it, i.e. begin work that undermines the prediction. This also inherently limits the ability to validate prospective prognostic predictions. We need to develop appropriate measures of assessing models as applied to present day patients while allowing for constant advances in treatment.

There is an inherent conflict between the need to keep a model simple enough to be integrated in clinical practice, yet be individualized enough to fulfill what clinicians want. One can manage some complexity (i.e. calculations) behind the scenes through computers, showing primarily simplified summary results (perhaps with further detail available for those who want it). However, the problem remains that individualized prognostic estimates will require data entry of multiple patient related, tumor related, environment related and treatment related data, which will take time and may render the model impractical for actual use.

It is clear that a clinically relevant model, applicable to specific patients in the present will be inherently messy and perhaps unappealing to statistical and methodologic purists. While we must have as solid a basis as possible, perhaps a focus on quantitative precision is not the right approach. We should recognize that the messy issues - deciding when to combine (or not) data from different sources, weighing the impact of prognostic factors defined in different datasets, extrapolating to the future, taking into account evolving changes - these issues are already being addressed every day as we exercise clinical judgment in caring for patients. Developing data-driven tools to augment clinical judgment is likely to be more readily achieved than a truly rigorous, precise model which is essentially designed to replace clinical judgment.

Transparent expression of the degree of uncertainty and the precision of applicability to a particular patient is a crucial feature of a system designed to enhance clinical judgment. This would promote appropriate interpretation of the prognostic estimates (i.e. how strongly they should be weighed). It would also indicate when the model is going beyond what the scientific basis will allow.

Typically clinicians (and patients) primarily think they want a specific prognostic prediction, (e.g. percent 5-year survival), tailored as much as possible to a specific patient. From this point of view, model calibration is most important. However, this is difficult to achieve, particularly when one moves from a retrospective definition of prognosis to a prospective prediction. On the other hand, for the purpose of guiding treatment decisions, it may be sufficient to know a patient's prognosis relative to other patients (i.e. discrimination). It has been much easier to assess discrimination and to show stable discriminatory transportability.[49] Many (but not all) of the challenges associated with prospective prediction will influence discrimination much less than calibration. A better understanding of what is really needed from a prognostic model will influence how this should be structured.

Where Do We Go from Here?

An ideal prognostic model would provide an estimate of specific outcomes for specific patients cared for at the present time. It would be grounded on factual data, which is inherently historical, but extrapolate into the future, which is inherently speculative. It would be sufficiently detailed to be reasonably applicable to an individual, but this must be balanced by being practical, having sufficient scientific grounding and providing a sufficiently reliable and specific estimate of prognosis. The uncertainties must be expressed along with the prognostic estimate in order to be interpreted correctly. The model would enhance (not replace) clinical decision making, which is the ability to weigh multiple factors and considerations to arrive at a management plan for a patient.

We should not be paralyzed by the complexity and formidable challenges inherent in developing such a prognostic model. We should focus on providing small incremental improvements to the way that clinical decision making is being practiced, not be overwhelmed by trying to achieve a perfect model. We need to develop a framework for the process of developing a clinically relevant system for prognostic prediction. We should break down the task into smaller components, and develop tools and approaches for each of these components. We must use as much rigor as possible to maintain a solid scientific basis for a system to estimate prognosis. We need a solid understanding of changing outcomes over time as well as issues associated with other types of transportability. We need to achieve a better understanding of exactly what information is needed to enhance our clinical decision making, and how to depict the limitations so that the data can be interpreted appropriately. We need to structure our thinking; we must combine data, statistical science, thoughtful extrapolation and ways of presenting data that can be integrated into clinical care and thus enhance clinical judgment. Hopefully this chapter will facilitate the ability to think more clearly about the many aspects and issues associated with this.

Development of a clinically useful prognostic model is a complex, challenging initiative that will take many years. Many issues will have to be addressed to build a framework. This framework must be flexible enough to permit continual evolution. A clear focus must be maintained on the actual user; this demands that the process is user friendly and provides measures that are practical and enhance clinical decision-making. To quote William Osler: "Medicine is a science of uncertainty and an art of probability."

References

1. Mahar A, Compton C, McShane L, et al. Refining prognosis in lung cancer. A report on the quality and relevance of clinical prognostic tools. *J Thorac Oncol* 2015;15(10):1576-1589.
2. Kyzas PA, Denaxa-Kyza D, Ioannidis JPA. Almost all articles on cancer prognostic markers report statistically significant results. *Eur J Cancer* 2007;43(17):2559-2579.
3. Riley RD, Sauerbrei W, Altman DG. Prognostic markers in cancer: the evolution of evidence from single studies to meta-analysis, and beyond. *Br J Cancer* 2009;100(8):1219-1229.
4. Detterbeck FC. Stage classification and prediction of prognosis: The difference between accountants and speculators. *J Thorac Oncol* 2013;8((7)):820-822.
5. Kerr K, Nicolson M. Prognostic factors in resected lung carcinomas. *EJC Supplements* 2013;11(2): 137-149.

6. Lindskog C, Edlund K, Sofia J, Mattsson M, Micke P. Immunohistochemistry-based prognostic bio-markers in NSCLC: novel findings on the road to clinical use? *Expert Rev Mol Diagn* 2015;15(4): 471-490.

7. Subramanian J, Simon R. Gene expression-based prognostic signatures in lung cancer: ready for clinical use? *J Natl Cancer Inst* 2010;102(7):464-474.

8. Mallett S, Royston P, Dutton S, Waters R, Altman D. Reporting methods in studies developing prog-nostic models in cancer: a review. *BMC Med* 2010;8(20):1-11.

9. Mallett S, Royston P, Waters R, Dutton S, Altman D. Reporting performance of prognostic models in cancer: a review. *BMC Medicine* 2010;8(21):1-11.

10. Bouwmeester W, Zuithoff N, Mallett S, et al. Reporting and methods in clinical prediction research: a systematic review. *PLoS Med* 2012;9(5):e1001221.

11. Dupuy A, Simon RM. Critical review of published microarray studies for cancer outcome and guide-lines on statistical analysis and reporting. *J Natl Cancer Inst* 2007;99(2):147-157.

12. Groome PA, Mahar A, McShane L, Halabi S, Pillsworth E, Compton C. The status of prognostic tools in oncology. *CA Cancer J Clin* 2016;in press.

13. Collins GS, De Groot JAH, Dutton S, et al. External validation of mutlitvariable prediction models: a systematic review of methodological conduct and reporting. *BMC Med Res Methodol* 2014;14(40):1-11.

14. Altman DG, Lausen B, Sauerbrei W, Schumacher M. Dangers of using "optimal" cutpoints in the evaluation of prognostic factors. *J Natl Cancer Inst* 1994;86(11):829-835.

15. McShane L, Altman D, Sauerbrei W, Taube S, Gion M, Clark GftSSotN-EWGoCD. Reporting recom-mendations for tumor MARKer prognostic studies (REMARK). *Nat Clin Pract Oncol* 2005;2(8):416-422.

16. Liang W, Zhang L, Jiang G, et al. Development and validation of a nomogram for predicting survival in patients with resected non–small-cell lung cancer. *J Clin Oncol* 2015;33(8):861-869.

17. Moons K, Altman D, Reitsma J, et al. Transparent reporting of a multivariable prediction model for individual prognosis or diagnosis (TRIPOD): explanation and elaboration. *Ann Intern Med* 2015;162:W1-W73.

18. Collins GS, Reitsma JB, Altman DG, Moons KGM. Transparent reporting of a multivariable predic-tion model for individual prognosis or diagnosis (TRIPOD): the TRIPOD Statement. *Ann Intern Med* 2015;162(1):55-63.

19. Chansky K, Sculier J, Crowley J, Giroux D, Van Meerbeeck J, Goldstraw P. The International Association for the Study of Lung Cancer Staging Project: prognostic factors and pathologic TNM stage in surgically managed non-small cell lung cancer. *J Thorac Oncol* 2009;4(7):792-801.

20. Dehing-Oberije C, Aerts H, Yu S, et al. Development and validation of a prognostic model using blood biomarker information for prediction of survival of non-small-cell lung cancer patients treated with combined chemotherapy and radiation or radiotherapy alone (NCT00181519, NCT00573040, and NCT00572325). *International journal of radiation oncology, biology, physics* 2011;81(2):360-368.

21. Dehing-Oberije C, Yu S, De Ruysscher D, et al. Development and external validation of prognostic model for 2-year survival of non-small-cell lung cancer patients treated with chemoradiotherapy. *International journal of radiation oncology, biology, physics* 2009;74(2):355-362.

22. Mandrekar S, Schild S, Hillman S, et al. A Prognostic Model for advanced stage nonsmall cell lung cancer. *Cancer* 2006;107(4):781-792.

23. Zhang K, Lai Y, Axelrod R, et al. Modeling the overall survival of patients with advanced-stage non-small cell lung cancer using data of routine laboratory tests. *Int J Cancer* 2015;136(2):382-391.

24. Sculier J-P, Chansky K, Crowley J, Van Meerbeeck JP, Goldstraw P. The impact of additional prog-nostic factors on survival and their relationship with the anatomical extent of disease expressed by the 6th Edition of the TNM classification of malignant tumors and the proposals for the 7th Edition. *J Thorac Oncol* 2008;3(5):457-466.

25. Akagi I, Okayama H, Schetter AJ, et al. Combination of protein coding and noncoding gene expression as a robust prognostic classifier in stage I lung adenocarcinoma. *Cancer Res* 2013;73(13):3821-3832.

26. Okayama H, Schetter AJ, Ishigame T, et al. The expression of four genes as a prognostic classifier for stage I lung adenocarcinoma in 12 independent cohorts. *Cancer Epidemiol Biomarkers Prev* 2014;23(12):2884-2894.

27. Pilotto S, Sperduti I, Novello S, et al. Risk stratification model for resected squamous-cell lung cancer patients according to clinical and pathological factors. *J Thorac Oncol* 2015;10(9):1341-1348.

28. Birim Ö, Kappetein AP, Waleboer M, et al. Long-term survival after non-small cell lung cancer surgery: development and validation of a prognostic model with a preoperative and postoperative mode. *J Thorac Cardiovasc Surg* 2006;132(3):491-498.

29. Robles AI, Arai E, Mathé EA, et al. An integrated prognostic classifier for Stage I lung adenocarcinoma based on mRNA, microRNA, and DNA methylation biomarkers. *J Thorac Oncol* 2015;10(7):1037-1048.

30. Zhang J, Gold KA, Lin HY, et al. Relationship between tumor size and survival in Non-Small-Cell Lung Cancer (NSCLC): an analysis of the Surveillance, Epidemiology, and End Results (SEER) registry. *J Thorac Oncol* 2015;10(4):682-690.

31. McGinn T, Guyatt G, Wyer P, Naylor C, Stiell I, Richardson W. Users'guides to the medical literature: XXII: how to use articles about clinical decision rules. Evidence-Based Medicine Working Group. *JAMA* 2000;284(1):79-84.

32. Concato J, Peduzzi P, Holford T, Feinstein A. Importance of events per independent variable in proportional hazards analysis I. Background, goals, and general strategy. *J Clin Epidemiol* 1995;48(12):1495-1501.

33. Peduzzi P, Concato J, Feinstein A, Holford T. Importance of events per independent variable in proportional hazards regression analysis II. Accuracy and precision of regression estimates. *J Clin Epidemiol* 1995;48(12):1503-1510.

34. Peduzzi P, Concato J, Kemper E, Holford T, Feinstein A. A simulation study of the number of events per variable in logistic regression analysis. *J Clin Epidemiol* 1996;49(12):1373-1379.

35. Austin P, Steyereberg E. Events per variable (EPV) and the relative performance of different strategies for estimating the out of sample validity of logistic regression models. *Stat Methods Med Res* Nov 19, 2014 2014:1-13.

36. Steyerberg E, Bleeker S, Moll H, Grobbee D, Moons K. Internal and external validation of predictive models: A simulation study of bias and precision in small samples. *J Clin Epidemiol* 2003;56(5):441-447.

37. Collins G, Ogundimu E, Altman D. Sample size considerations for the external validation of a multivariable prognostic model: a resampling study. *Statist Med* 2016;35(2):214-226.

38. Vergouwe Y, Steyerberg E, Eijkemans M, Habbema J. Substantial effective sample sizes were required for external validation studies of predictive logistic regression models. *J Clin Epidemiol* 2005;58(5):475-483.

39. Royston P, Altman DG. External validation of a Cox prognostic model: principles and methods. *BMC Med Res Methodol* 2013;13:33.

40. Debray T, Vergouwe Y, Koffijberg H, Nieboer D, Steyerberg E, Moons K. A new framework to enhance the interpretation of external validation studies of clinical prediction models. *J Clin Epidemiol* 2015;68(3):279-289.

41. O'Hurley G, Sjöstedt E, Rahman A, et al. Garbage in, garbage out: A critical evaluation of strategies used for validation of immunohistochemical biomarkers. *Mol Oncol* 2014;8(4):783-798.

42. Howat W, Lewis A, Jones P, et al. Antibody validation of immunohistochemistry for biomarker discovery: recommendations of a consortium of academic and pharmaceutical based histopathology researchers. *Methods* 2014;70(1):34-38.

43. Janssens A, Ioannidis J, Van Duijn C, Little J, Khoury M. Strengthening the reporting of genetic risk prediction studies: The GRIPS statement. *Eur J Clin Invest* 2011;41(9):1004-1009.

44. Janssens A, Ioannidis J, Bedrosian S, et al. Strengthening the reporting of genetic risk prediction studies (GRIPS): explanation and elaboration. *Eur J Clin Invest* 2011;41(9):1010-1035.

45. Little J, Higgins JPT, Ioannidis JPA, et al. STrengthening the REporting of Genetic Association Studies (STREGA)— An Extension of the STROBE Statement. *PLoS Med* 2009;6(2):e22.

46. Swanton C, Govindan R. Clinical implications of genomic discoveries in lung cancer. *N Engl J Med* 2016;374(19):1864-1873.

47. Kattan M, Hess K, Amin M, et al. American Joint Committee on Cancer acceptance criteria for inclusion of risk models for individualized prognosis in the practice of precision medicine. *CA Cancer J Clin* 2016;66(5):370-4.

48. Altman DG, Vergouwe Y, Royston P, Moons KGM. Prognosis and prognostic research: validating a prognostic model. *BMJ* 2009;338:b605.

49. Detterbeck F, Chansky K, Groome P, et al. The IASLC Lung Cancer Staging Project: methodology and validation used in the development of proposals for revision of the stage classification of non-small cell lung cancer in the forthcoming (8th) edition of the TNM classification of lung cancer. *J Thorac Oncol* 2016;11: 1433-1446.

50. Detterbeck FC. Maintaining aim at a moving target. *J Thorac Oncol* 2011;6(3):417-422.

51. Morgensztern D, Ng SH, Gao F, Govindan R. Trends in stage distribution for patients with non-small cell lung cancer: a National Cancer Database survey. *J Thorac Oncol* 2010;5(1):29-33.

52. Chee KG, Nguyen DV, Brown M, Gandara DR, Wun T, Lara PN, Jr. Positron emission tomography and improved survival in patients with lung cancer: the Will Rogers phenomenon revisited. *Arch Intern Med* 2008;168(14):1541-1549.

53. Morgensztern D, Waqar S, Subramanian J, Gao F, Govindan R. Improving survival for stage IV non-small cell lung cancer: a surveillance, epidemiology, and end results survey from 1990 to 2005. *J Thorac Oncol* 2009;4(12):1524-1529.

54. Janssen KJM, Vergouwe Y, Kalkman CJ, Grobbee DE, Moons KGM. A simple method to adjust clinical prediction models to local circumstances. *Can J Anaesth* 2009;56(3):194-201.

55. van Houwelingen HC. Validation, calibration, revision and combination of prognostic survival models. *Stat Med* 2000;19(24):3401-3415.

56. Altman DG, Royston P. What do we mean by validating a prognostic model? *Stat Med* 2000;19(4): 453-473.

57. Detterbeck FC. Stage classification and prognosis: an intersection of medicine, quantum physics and religion? *Thorax* 2011;66(11):1016-1017.

58. Reilly B, Evans A. Translating clinical research into clinical practice: impact of using prediction rules to make decisions. *Ann Intern Med* 2006;144(3):201-209.

59. Moons K, de Groot J, Bouwmeester W, et al. Critical appraisal and data extraction for systematic reviews of prediction modelling studies: the CHARMS checklist. *PLoS Medicine* 2014;11(10):e1001744.

Index